COLOUR THERAPY

Also in this series

HOW TO BE A MEDIUM
J. Donald Walters
HOW TO DEVELOP YOUR ESP
Zak Martin
MEDITATION: THE INNER WAY
Naomi Humphrey
PRACTICAL VISUALIZATION
Chris Odle
UNDERSTANDING ASTRAL PROJECTION
Anthony Martin
UNDERSTANDING THE CHAKRAS
Peter Rendel
UNDERSTANDING THE I CHING
Tom Riseman
UNDERSTANDING NUMEROLOGY
D. Jason Cooper
UNDERSTANDING PALMISTRY
Mary Anderson
UNDERSTANDING REINCARNATION
J. H. Brennan
UNDERSTANDING RUNES
Michael Howard

COLOUR THERAPY

The application of colour for healing, diagnosis
and well-being

by

Mary Anderson

THE AQUARIAN PRESS

This edition 1990
First published as *Colour Healing* 1975

© MARY ANDERSON 1979

British Library Cataloguing in Publication Data

Anderson, Mary
Colour therapy.
1. Medicine. Chromotherapy
I. Title II. Anderson , Mary. Colour healing
615.831

ISBN 1-85538-010-2

*The Aquarian Press is part of the Thorsons Publishing Group,
Wellingborough, Northamptonshire, NN8 2RQ, England*

Printed in Great Britain by William Collins Sons & Co. Ltd,
Glasgow

1 3 5 7 9 10 8 6 4 2

CONTENTS

INTRODUCTION

Gradually, since the end of the war, colour has been coming back into our lives, taking up the place it held in Regency times after its long eclipse under the Victorians.

Contemporary colour is bold and bright — perhaps this is the defiant gesture of a frightened world where the Bomb looms large and our breakfast cornflakes take second place to each new horror revealed in newsprint, or perhaps it is that we are so uninhibited now. Whatever the reason, the new colours are here; browns, greys and creams have been ousted by bold, true colours. The reds are very red, the blues are exquisite, ranging from a very pale pastel blue to indigo, the greens delight and soothe us and the yellows are bold, having caught a little bit of sunshine on the way.

Colour expresses the way we think and then reacts back on us from our surroundings, either raising or lowering our spirits. It is evident that the richness and diversity of colour which we see around us at the present time reflects the thinking of a more joyful, open and honest age than the one just passed.

Past civilizations such as those influenced by Byzantine art were fortunate in that they were surrounded by wonderful colours, including stripes and chequered effects, which lifted the spirits and encouraged people to feel happy and glad to be alive. Today, especially in our cities, we have grey built-up buildings, all very similar in colour (or maybe one should say 'non-colour'). People feel devitalized and dispirited by the sameness of it all. Were there more colour in our everyday surroundings, life would be more cheerful and interesting.

In great cities like London there is very little room for gardens, which bring in the soothing colour green, an antidote to the high-powered tension of the professional districts. Fortunately, there are some parks, such as St James's Park, Regents Park and Kensington Gardens. They are essential to the physical and mental well-being of those who live and work in the city. The cities in tropical countries, however, present their natives and visitors with more vibrantly coloured buildings. It is possible that Prince Charles has in mind the colours of the buildings he has been criticizing recently as well as their shape. Maybe he too is subconsciously affected by the dullness of colours used in buildings which so many of us have to pass every day of our lives.

We can see how important colour is in the home. More and more we seek to express ourselves and our attitudes to life by the colours which we use in our homes. What a difference colours make to our walls, how decorative wallpaper can be and how important the contribution which pictures can make to our rooms! The curtains play their part too in expressing our individual message to the world. Wherever we see a house painted pink, yellow or white, the whole street is cheered by this expression of colour.

Colour can be used constructively, that is the right colour in the right situation, or negatively and out of context. Red in a dining room, for instance, is not appropriate since you need a peaceful green/blue/pink area to enjoy, assimilate and digest your food and to find pleasure in the companionship which is offered.

Psychologically, we are much affected by colour. We are cheered by vivid colours, while drab colours give us a correspondingly dull feeling. Red, for example, is a warming colour. The warmth of an open fire is unexcelled, for although we can get a more even warmth through other forms of heating, the sight of the burning red coals affects us psychologically, and we associate a real home with a fire glowing there, ready and waiting for us to return. Even more friendly and warming is the heat given out by a peat or log fire, with its country associations, implying peace and security against the elements.

Colour plays, therefore, a more important part in our lives than we are consciously aware of. It influences our actions and reactions. Colours, wherever they are found — of clothes, on walls, in advertisements — are always conveying their subtle messages to us below the level of conscious awareness. Our minds and bodies understand these messages, for they hold out promises of fulfilment to us. Some speak of relaxation, some offer a stimulus to action. These subtle suggestions are with us all our lives and mostly we are obedient to their instructions.

We are continually seeing advertisements for various washing powders and in experiments it has been found that the colour of the packet has a great influence on the sales of the powder. In one experiment three different packets were tested. One was yellow, the second blue and the third a mixture of the two colours. The majority vote was for the powder from the carton with the mixture of blue and yellow. The reason given for this was that the powder from the yellow carton was found to be too strong, the powder from the blue carton too weak and the one from the blue and yellow carton just right. The interesting thing was that the powder in all three packets was the same. People's reaction to it was purely psychological, based upon their unconscious understanding of the quality of the colour on the packet of detergent. For instance, yellow is a stimulating colour, so the message of the yellow carton was, 'this is too strong,' while the message of the blue carton was 'this is too weak,' for blue is a cool, restful colour, bringing with it a sense of peace. The *combination* of these two colours on the cover of the third carton sent the subliminal message, 'this carton has a balanced and effective content. It is just right.'

From this you can see how very important the right colour tone is for the advertiser of a product in his bid to maximize sales. For instance, suppose a publisher has a book on his list of forthcoming titles on *love*. He would be extremely unwise to offer a *black* jacket even if there were other embellishments on it. Black is the negation of colour itself; it expresses the idea of extinction. Its message is *no*, you have reached your limits. It is the opposite of *white*, whose message is *yes*, go ahead, there are no limits. Black then represents a giving up, a renunciation of desirable things. Hardly the right message on the jacket of a book on love. Needless to say, such a book would have a very small sale and would very soon be out of print. Light, subtle colours such as pale pink, pale blue and yellow, or just a white jacket with a heart in the centre would be more appropriate and achieve the purpose of circulation.

Notice how it is that sugar is sold in packets with blue and pink motifs. We associate these colours with sweetness and it is certain that if sugar were sold in green packets it would languish on the shelves.

It is interesting to note that fashion designers, who have to keep a very sharp eye on which colours will be in fashion this year or next, draw their own conclusions as to their client's character by the predominating colours their wardrobes contain. If red and yellow predominate, then the owner is extrovert, exciting, impulsive and changeable, while if more sober colours like grey and black predominate, then the owner is much more self-disciplined and cautious, prefers more traditional, suave and subtle clothes and is likely to be less extroverted.

People in general do react in similar fashion to various

colours. Blue for instance, has a calming effect upon us. Red is stimulating — it is the colour of blood and in earlier times when mankind lived more primitively by the hunt, at the end of a good day's hunt blood has flowed and food had been obtained. Life could continue for the tribe. Green represents nature, its leafy fastnesses providing shelter for animal life, including our own. Yellow is stimulating, acting with mankind's deep worship of the sun as the giver of life. At the rising of the sun, man was reminded of the duties and pleasures of the day before him and arose to greet the new day.

Imagine the exciting influences of the bright coloured lights used in discos. The movement, taken with the music, is all very stimulating.

Not only do colours influence us psychologically and emotionally, they also affect us physically. It is for this reason that it is possible to use colour to heal.

Red, we know, is exciting to us psychologically, but it also has a physical influence. It causes our blood pressure to rise if we are confronted with it for any length of time. Remember when the bull fighter wishes to rouse the bull to action, a red cloak is drawn provocatively across the bull's angle of vision until the desired result is achieved. Where both man and animal are concerned the pulse and respiration rate are also speeded up when red is the predominant colour for any length of time. With colour there is always an answer to a problem like high blood pressure and the answer in this case is Blue. Blue has a cool, calming effect and causes the blood pressure to fall. Pulse and respiration rate slow down too.

Professor Max Lüscher has evolved a system of colour analysis which can pinpoint a great number of characteristics, both psychological and physiological, from the colours patients like or dislike. Patients are shown various colours and colour combinations which they are asked to place in order of preference. The Lüscher Colour Test is in book form and can be used by lay people or therapists. It is published by Jonathan Cape. Cards of different colours are included in the book for use in testing. The Lüscher Colour Test is comprehensive; apparently the only thing which cannot be ascertained by this method is whether you are intelligent or not. But it can determine whether you are aggressive, confident, insecure, placid or ambitious and also reveals emotional attitudes. It can show whether a patient is sensual, frigid, trustworthy, responsible or over-indulgent and if he is stable emotionally, overreacting to the point of suicide, or overworking in a compulsive sort of way, perhaps even running the risk of a heart attack.

The full test is really complex and is contained in the book mentioned earlier. When the test is done at the Institute of Psychodiagnostic Medicine at Basle in Switzerland, where Professor Lüscher evolved his system, blood pressure, pulse rate and respiration are checked, something it is not possible to do if you are testing yourself. However, if you are a therapist or a lay person you can learn to analyse yourself and others quite effectively. The test is, of course, used quite extensively by psychologists and psychiatrists.

Research on the part of psychologists, designers, marketing and advertising experts has given us a pretty good idea of the colour of your personality from your colour choice. On the back of this book there are 10 bands of colour. Pick the colour you like best:

If you have picked *yellow*: You have an interesting and stimulating personality. You like to be active and involved in whatever is going on. Lively and vital, you can cope well with life's challenges.

If you have picked *white*: You have a positive, well balanced and optimistic personality. You are confident that you can cope with anything that comes your way.

If you have picked *red*: You are impulsive, excitable and active. You like things to happen quickly when you want them to do so. You like to be the best in everything you do.

You may be a bit insensitive to the feelings of other people.

If you have picked *blue*: You could be called a bit laid back. You do not like to be rushed and take your pleasures languidly. You may be a bit lazy. However, you like security and will work for this. You do like time to yourself.

If you have picked *green*: You are a cautious person and not inclined to trust others easily. You are an observer of life, but do not wish to get involved more than you have to. A quiet life suits you best.

If you have picked *violet*: Yours is a sensitive, compassionate nature so you can be easily imposed upon and should be careful to pick friends who are as sensitive as you are yourself. To be happy, work where you feel needed.

If you have picked *purple*: You are interested in the best of everything, including among your friends those from the top drawer. Lesser mortals do not interest you or enter into your scheme of things except where necessary. Slightly arrogant.

If you have picked *grey*: You are very much a one-man band. Many people may get the impression you are self-sufficient. You keep yourself under excellent control and to yourself.

If you have picked *brown*: A lover of the best things life has to offer, you are a sensuous type appreciating good food, fine wine and the best company in elegant surroundings with minions indulging your tasteful whims.

If you have picked *black*: You lack confidence in yourself and your own ability to handle life efficiently. It may be you have a little way to go towards maturity, but once you make progress in this direction you'll be fine.

You can of course use this with your friends, each one making their own pick.

The sayings, 'seeing red' and 'feeling blue', 'green with jealousy' and 'black with rage', all relate to actual changes which take place in the colours of our own electro-magnetic field due to changes in our emotions. This electro-magnetic field which surrounds everything, not only the human being, is often referred to as the aura. It is quite easy to assure yourself of the truth of this assertion by a little experiment. Ask a friend to stand with a light behind him and against a light-coloured wall. It is often easier to see the aura by not looking at it directly, but by concentrating on some point on the person's body, like the end of his nose — embarrassing perhaps, so try his tie instead — then gradually you will see the faint glow around the head first and then around the whole body. To some people the aura appears to be white at first, but with practice the colours will appear.

This aura, which is usually visible to sensitives, is often the means by which the colour/healer diagnoses. The affected organ or part will show a dark or discoloured mark in the aura over the place where the disharmony exists. As each colour has a different vibration, colour healing is really operating on exactly similar lines to any other form of healing. In the same way that the doctor hopes that his pills will adjust the disharmony in the vibrational rate, so the contact or colour healer hopes for the same effect. The chemical imbalance of the body — which shows itself as a disease — may be corrected by chemical means or by means of the fine rays sent out in colour healing.

The colour healer, having diagnosed the condition, or in some instances having been told by the patient and checked this by his own observations, will proceed to apply remedial colours where there is a deficiency, or contrasting colours where there is an excess. He may do this by applying the rays of different coloured lamps or simply by directing the invisible rays which swirl around and through us day and night. He acts as a selector and conveyor of power, which he passes on to the patient. Some patients feel the application of the rays, others feel nothing, but all must benefit, although some more than others.

Taken all in all, colour is an integral part of our lives. It brings us joy, gaiety, and — when we need it — healing. Visible and invisible, it affects us powerfully, for in it we live and have our being.

CHAPTER ONE

THE SCIENTIFIC BACKGROUND

We are all affected by colour in our everyday lives, but what is colour? The shortest definition which the dictionary gives us is that it is a quality of light. In an everyday sense we accept that our environment is subject to fluctuations in this quality of light; the day may be sunny, or drab and wet, for example, and there are many variations in between these two poles. This is due to the rays or vibrations which are continually playing around and through everything in the world, although in most instances we cannot see them with our physical sight.

However, there is an inner significance behind the outer show and to the occultist and to many colour healers there is an age-old belief that in the truest sense *colour is life* and that the play of colour which manifests as light is the visible expression of the Divine Mind, of the one life principle in the form of light waves.

The ancient Egyptians knew of the power and influence of colour and in their great temples, such as Karnak and Thebes, there were *colour halls* where research into the use of colour and colour healing were practised.

System of Colour Science

Manuscripts from these early times show that in India, China and Egypt, the healer priests had a complete system of colour science, based on the law of correspondence between the sevenfold nature of man and the sevenfold division of the solar spectrum. Therefore the fundamental laws and principles governing the cosmic energy we know as colour have always been present in the Ancient Wisdom teachings for teachers and healers of all ages. However, modern research, physics, and metaphysics are all uncovering the wisdom of the ancients regarding the use of colour in healing, and we will view the matter first of all from the more orthodox angle, where doctors and scientists have interested themselves in research into the use of nature's finer forces for the effective healing of many ailments, and as a result have actually used colour therapeutically with success.

Given that disease is a want of harmony in the system, the idea behind colour healing, or chromotherapy, is to restore bodily imbalance through the application of beams of coloured light to the body.

Although colour healing, like many other sciences being revived today, bases its roots in the past, in modern times interest in it really began with experiments done on plants by Robert Hunt, whose book, *Researches on Light In Its Chemical Relations*, described the influences on plant growth of selected applications of light. The first book written on the use of colour for therapeutic purposes, entitled *Blue and Red Light, or Light and Its Rays as Medicine*, by Dr S. Pancoast, was published in 1877. Basically it dealt with the use of the stimulating red and the soothing blue rays, contrasting their effects on the human body.

The following year Dr Edwin D. Babbitt published his monumental work *The Principles of Light and Colour* describing the effects of the different colours of the spectrum and their use as healing agents. However, it was a Hindu scientist by the name of D. P. Ghadiali who discovered the scientific principles which explain why and how the different coloured rays have various therapeutic effects on the organism. In 1933, after years of research, Ghadiali published *The Spectro Chromemetry Encyclopaedia*, a master work on colour therapy. He worked and taught in the USA, developing many types of colour lamps.

Ghadiali's Theories

The theories developed here come from Ghadiali's work. He stated that colours represent chemical potencies in higher octaves of vibration.

For each organism and system of the body there is a particular colour that stimulates and another that inhibits the work of that organ or system.

By knowing the action of the different colours upon the different organs and systems of the body, one can apply the correct colour that will tend to balance the action of any organ or system that has become abnormal in its functioning or condition.

The process of living in a healthy state involves a proper balance within the body of all the colour energies. When this balance is disturbed disease results, and if the imbalance becomes too great, death occurs. The aim of the science of colour healing is to combat disease by restoring the normal balance of colour energies within the body.

The earth and all its inhabitants obtain energy from the sun's rays — all elements known on earth are found in the sun, as shown by spectroscopic analysis. The sun's rays bring us the energies of every known element, from which all chemical combinations are made. White light contains the energies of all elements and chemicals found in the sun.

The sun is constantly pouring white light energy into the atmosphere, thus 'charging' this atmosphere with the different types of energy necessary to sustain life.

The Auric Body

Man has an auric body surrounding and interpenetrating his physical body. One of the functions of the aura is to absorb the white light energy from the atmosphere and split it into component colour energies, which then flow to the different parts of the body to vitalize them. Research indicates that it is probable that the effects noted from the use of colour therapy occur through the action of colour rays upon the auric body, which in turn influences the physical body.

In the human individual there are two basic processes at work all the time, namely anabolism and catabolism. The former is a building up and repairing process, while the latter is the opposite and deals with the elimination of toxic or waste products from the body. Good health can only be maintained if a proper balance is kept between the two processes of anabolism and catabolism, which together represent metabolism.

Primary Colours in Chromotherapy

Ghadiali found that the red ray is the colour of construction, that is, it maintains the number of red blood cells in the body and stimulates the liver, whilst the violet ray, which activates the spleen, is the colour of destruction or catabolism. He discovered that the spleen destroyed the older red blood cells and produced the white blood cells that combat bacteria.

In the spectrum, red — which stimulates the liver activity — is at one end of the visible spectrum of light, while violet — which stimulates splenic activity — is at the other end of the visible spectrum of light. The central or balancing colour of the spectrum of visible light is green, which is the colour that activates or encourages the activity of the pituitary gland, long known to be a master gland and controller of the other glands, and so affecting the action of every part of the body. Ghadiali said, 'We have come a long way, but we have now found our balancer for the body and it is green, the central body of the visible spectrum of light which fosters balance in the body between the opposing actions of the liver and the spleen, between anabolism and catabolism, and this is accomplished through the medium of the pituitary gland.'

From the foregoing it will be understood that Ghadiali found red, green and violet to be the primary colours in chromotherapy. Red, yellow and blue, he said, were the primary colours when working with pigments, but light rays follow different laws from those that apply to the mixing of pigments. Ghadiali tested out many colour theories over decades, but these were the only ones proved right by extensive experiments.

You may ask: Why colour healing, when there are so many other methods? The answer is that chromotherapy has many advantages. Ghadiali himself states, 'Thousands of drugs are used in medical practice,' and asks, 'Is it wise to dump so many into the human body when they are not included in the natural composition of the body?' He also said, '... Chemicals are life potencies; their atoms have attractions and repulsions, and to endeavour to introduce haphazard inorganic metals into an organic machine is like feeding a baby with steel tacks to make it strong.'

Another point made by Ghadiali in this respect is that deviation in the body above or below its normal percentage is a prime cause of illness, but doctors often unwittingly increase the imbalance, or reverse it to the opposite side, with their remedies, hence the many drug-induced illnesses.

Unreliable Drugs

Drugs can be unreliable, since people react variously to different drugs. Witness the many people allergic to penicillin and allied drugs. In contrast, chromotherapy leaves no harmful residues which the body has to work hard to eliminate. Chromotherapy does not treat symptoms, it goes to the root of the imbalance. Many of the illnesses to which man is heir have their root in the auric body and this can be seriously damaged by strong drugs. Chromotherapy uses the type of remedy which most closely matches the constituents of the auric bodies. It is the premise of chromotherapy that by giving colour ray treatment instead of drugs, a constructive result can be obtained without any accompanying destructive effect.

In this respect it is interesting to note that for some reason the medical profession use the vibratory light spectrum just below and just above the visible light band, but are slow in acknowledging the healing properties of the visible light spectrum. Actually, of course, both infra-red and ultra-violet rays cause tissue damage if used to any sizeable extent, while the most which can occur by the use of an incorrect colour from the visible light spectrum, or if too long an exposure is given, is a temporary accentuation of a functional disorder.

In fact where both lay and medical therapists have used colour therapy they have been well pleased with the results.

Going Back to the Beginning

We have just seen how in the opinion of esoteric teachers today we have to understand light and use it with more awareness. Theo Gimbel expresses this very well in his work *Man: The Healer Through Colour*, in which he shows how to help man today it is necessary to go back to the origins of matter and the various stages through which the planet developed. The stages he states are as follows: darkness, light, colour, form. Light and darkness create colour. Colour sinking down to lower vibratory rates manifests as sound. This creates form and crystals, which, as we are beginning to rediscover, are original sound forms. Colour into sound happens as a polarity action such as breathing in man, plant and animal. This is the beginning of time, the womb of creation.

Out of the original complementary energies of dark and light arises the third, which is colour. Colour is the subtle interaction between darkness (feminine) and light (masculine). It is interesting to note that as early as 1810 Johann Wolfgang von Goethe wrote a most useful book on the theory of colour.

After the formation of colour, the next step in the development of the planet was the swing into sound, then the intensification of colour, from which came hearing. Sound can actually produce beautiful forms and shapes. Musical sound can shift sands on a flat surface into various patterns.

The Gospel of St John starts with the words: 'In the beginning was the Word and the Word was with God — and the word was God ...' St John makes it very clear that the point of impact of the invisible on the field of inert matter produces living matter, raising this to actual life, and visible man, animal, plant and stone appear. This then is a tremendous evolutionary step. Into matter is implanted the living God who can raise this matter to eternal life.

Unfortunately, it is man's failure to continue this work effectively which causes disease.

Having descended into matter, the future must be the ascent of man, and this can be done by recapturing a vision of what is possible for him, what is his true destiny. This can by done by love and by offering healing where it is needed. Colour is the healer. It is interesting to note that in near death experiences, the message of those who return from beyond is very simple, and the same in practically all recorded instances: that love is the most necessary thing for the world today to heal its wounds, and in order for people to make progress they should try and advance their knowledge and understanding. Now we need to find again our lost vision which has been obscured by gaining material things such as television, cars, computers, etc. These do not contribute to man's true dignity or his way to the stars.

To gain more understanding we need to research into all the vibrations of the various kingdoms of the earth — the human, animal, plant and stone — and not only into the known vibrations, but also into those relatively unknown, those which are invisible, such as the sound and aura of nature.

Everything which we can see has an aura around it, an electrical force field, which some people can see; and Kirlian photography makes visible its etheric radiation. This is seen as a narrow band around plants, animals and man. Its discovery was due to the work of two Russian scientists, Semyon and Valentina Kirlian. In order to carry out this technique a high-voltage generator uses a photographic film. What becomes visible in this way is not the actual aura, but the etheric sheath outlining the body.

Kirlian photography is now being used to diagnose disease and also to check the quality of our food. This comes up clearly under a Kirlian photograph. There is a tremendous difference between food radiating goodness and that which is dead. For our lives we are all dependent on electro-magnetic radiation — more specifically the radiation of light — for our sustenance.

It is interesting to see that as man is gripped by computermania communication becomes more and more difficult. First of all physically on the roads we can hardly move, for we are all jammed up in our wonderful cars. These would indeed be wonderful if they had not proliferated to clutter up the whole environment and so make it really difficult to move around. Probably in the next move to clear our space, people will have to take to the air, or even go the moon, emigrate from the planet itself, for our earth is becoming too small for the number of people who want to incarnate at this time. It's all so exciting, people cannot wait to come back here and battle their way through again.

Relying as we do though on computers and television to keep life moving, in other words on man's creations, things can grind to a halt and there can be a total breakdown of communication, which can make progress impossible. This is being made even more certain by computer viruses, and people who deliberately break in on computer data are another problem.

Even so, we are in touch with wherever our thoughts travel. If we think of the sun or any of the planets we are immediately in touch with their energies. The priest-philosopher Teilhard de Chardin tells us that man is himself the sole means of procuring a full and total image of the future of mankind, and that he needs to recooperate with all the terrestial and celestial energies. When we look at life from the narrow angle of our personal lives and the small things that go on around us we limit both ourselves and mankind. We have a million things to discover or rediscover, and we have some very difficult tasks which cannot be accomplished in one or even two or three lifetimes, as we contemplate the magnitude of the possibilities for the future of the world, of all the worlds. A far grander vision faces us. Sometime we have to take up the challenge; the door is only slightly open now and we are beginning to see a new way forward. The way of ascent is possible as awareness grows and the seeds which have been planted come to fruition.

CHAPTER TWO

THE AURA, CHAKRAS, AND SUBTLE BODIES

In the Introduction, the electro-magnetic field which surrounds everything and which is known as the aura was mentioned in relation to healing and diagnosis.

It may not come amiss at this point to look into the build up of this aura. Before the birth of a child there are of course energy exchanges between the two parents and the third party, the child, who needs to come into contact with the earth.

The etheric is the blueprint upon which the physical is built, and this includes the various systems, the nervous system, the circulatory system, the brain and the heart. All these with their different colours are built up into a lovely aura which expresses the new baby at the completion of the pregnancy. All this growth is overseen by the pineal and pituitary glands. So many visible and even more invisible, spiritual changes occur in order to allow the new little one to take its place in the world. Nothing, however, is perfect and the aura will have its weaknesses and imperfections which open the gates to diseases in later life. Known homeoepathically as miasms, or inherited tendencies to disease, they can be detected by means of a pendulum used by a properly-trained psychic. They can then be treated either by colour healing or some other type of healing. Very often these 'lacks' can be treated simply by taking the required vitamins or minerals, or alternatively by cutting out some item of diet to which we may be allergic.

Very often quite simple adjustments to our way of life or to our diet can make a very big difference to health and happiness.

Seeing the Aura

While the existence of the aura had always been known to occultists and clairvoyants, it was not until Dr W. J. Kilner of St Thomas's Hospital, London, accepted that it existed and began to experiment to make it visible to the human eye, that the ordinary person could see it. Dr Kilner developed the 'dicyanin screen', a lens painted with a coal-tar dye. This has a remarkable effect upon vision and enables the eye to perceive the ultra-violet range.

Medicine was in an exciting and progressive period when the young Dr Kilner joined the staff of St Thomas's Hospital in the late 1800s. Contemporary researchers were Professor W. K. Röntgen, discoverer of the X-ray, Dr Braid, whose work on the use of hypnosis is well known, and a German scientist, Karl von Reichenbach, who was publishing his findings on what he called 'odic force', a luminous emanation surrounding the body. At the same time — in the USA — Dr Edwin D. Babbitt was engaged on *The Principles of Light and Colour*. Great forces were advancing the scope of healing into fields hitherto forgotten, except by the few who had inherited the wisdom of a vanished epoch.

When Dr Kilner published his book, *The Human Atmosphere*, it was not well-received by orthodoxy. He was laughed at and discredited. However, he did not give up his experiments with the dicyanin screen and continued until the First World War cut off his supply of dicyanin, which was produced in Germany. Using the Kilner screen and working within the ultra-violet range, the aura can be seen as an inner band outlining the body, while a second band of almost vaporous light extends away from the body.

Through use of the Kilner screen the eyes become sensitized and so the aura may be seen as a grey-blue emanation. The most orthodox doctor could avail himself of this screen and so examine the condition of his patient, for the aura shows a dark or discoloured mark over the affected area.

Thoughts Are All Around Us

Thoughts also form part of our environment every day of our lives. First of all we have our own thoughts — hopefully we make these positive and forward-looking. Then we have to receive the thoughts of all those others with whom we share our lives. Sometimes we only brush against these people momentarily, but we are still assailed by their thoughts. Apparently a camera has been invented which enables us to photograph thoughts. Interestingly enough, thoughts take various shapes. Thoughts of love bring pleasant shapes; those of hatred or jealousy are ugly. Thought is radiated from the mental body and has a filmy, vaporous appearance. It also shows the various colour tones of its essential nature. We dispatch our thoughts to the corners of the earth, and happy is the person on the receiving end of some positive, light-bearing thoughts.

The human being is like a radio. It receives as well as broadcasts messages. The distance a thought can travel really depends upon its strength, whether for good or ill. We are often being told that it is useless to pray with our lips in a habitual prattle without really thinking what we are asking. For our prayers to be answered we have to keep our concentration going, so that our desires may be taken up by the powers that be and realized on earth. If we wish to send thoughts of love we need to concentrate upon what we are doing and it is as well to colour our thoughts. For love we would use pink, as it is a colour which is generally accepted as being the colour of love. Other colours could be any pale pastel shades. People then can be healers and destroyers in their own right through their thought power. You will find some people really suck the life out of you. These people are unconscious vampires. They may be weak, sick and/or negative. After an hour in their presence you will feel depleted. This is because they have been drawing on your force. They go away feeling really great, their step is bouncy and their heads are held high, but their negativity will soon reassert itself unless its cause is attacked at root. In order to protect yourself from these psychic vampires cover yourself in the golden light of the sun so that your aura is strong enough to withstand the unconscious depletion from the sick person. Remember though that these people are not conscious of taking your energy, they need it and do not realize they are refurbishing themselves at someone else's expense.

Quite apart from this we all live in a sea of thought. Thoughts are around us all the time, and the pleasanter they are the better off we are. When absent healing is being sent, radiantly-coloured thoughts are directed to the patient and the effect is nearly always a change of feeling which brings with it renewed strength and positive courage. In a general sense we can all improve or deplete the psychic atmosphere.

Successful healing demonstrates that thought power gets results. Conversely, it must be true that evil thoughts have a depleting and destructive effect. For example, the power of the witch doctor to heal or destroy has been demonstrated too often to be dismissed as mumbo jumbo by Western doctors who have witnessed these events. The death of the person who has been cursed is taken for granted in some African societies.

What wonderful results we would get if this thought power was organized, particularly with the right colour visualization. The very fact that the thought power of a single individual can have such results points to the powerful force which a group of people could have if applied to a worthy cause.

On the other hand we can see how dangerous it is for a group of people or a nation to operate from an evil thought base. This was demonstrated to the world during the Second World War when the twisted mind of the leader of the German race led the German nation into actions of such horror against the Jews and other victims of his spite that the whole world was totally repelled and disgusted. This hate power does not go away in spite of the lessons which the world learnt throughout that war and after. We still have the same sort of hate being spewed forth by fundamentalists in the Middle East. This time the hate is directed not so much at the Jews (although this could arise at any time), but against the Americans, the British and Europeans in general. The British Isles suffers the hate of one part of Ireland towards the other and towards the British. All these evil thoughts based in the hatred of one human being against the other, basically in the name of religion.

People need not be influenced by evil or selfish thought forms. It is useful to remember that like goes to like and we need not fear negative thoughts, unless we harbour corresponding base thoughts which can, of course, draw evil thoughts our way. A spring cleaning of these can eliminate such a disaster.

Strong desires are expressed in strong thought forms which work to achieve those things we think we need. However, we should never send out injurious thoughts regarding another person. In esoteric law it is stated that the wish acts as a boomerang and the evil thought is projected back to him who sent it.

There must be a tremendous thought bank of ideas relating to all man's creativity on this planet. This must be the universal mind and we all have access to it. For those of you who meditate, the solution to a problem or an idea for a new project will often come to you during or after your meditation or when you are engrossed in doing something quite different. How often an idea will come like a bolt out of the blue to clarify a situation. Many writers tell us, 'we did not write the book, it wrote itself. The ideas just came to us, we just wrote them down.' This suggests that ideas once sent out and not realized have quite a powerful desire to be expressed and will try to realize themselves through someone who can help them to do so. In fact, we seem to be channels perhaps, rather than creators — some people just express some ideas better than others, as their background is conducive to their doing so. In theory we could all catch the elusive thoughts from the universal thought bank, but in practice only a certain few are successful. It seems that all time is here with us now in the present. As we work upon it and realize its ideas, we bring ourselves into harmony with all the ideas stored in the Universal Mind from all eternity.

As this is a book about colour healing it is wonderful to note that for those who need better health, the same principle applies. All healing thoughts exist in the ether today, and it is possible to draw to oneself the correct healing colours or to have these drawn for you by a colour therapist.

What one can say with truth is that everything we need to be whole and healthy already exists. Strength and health already exist — they are there waiting to be called upon by the individual. Christ said, 'Ask and you shall receive.' People either do not know this or do not believe it. It is not difficult to put yourself in tune with the universal principle of health and with that particular colour vibration which will do the healing job for you.

For this to work with you, you have to clear your mind

of all doubt and prejudice. Then ask for health or for a particular healing, relax on the demand and await the response, which you can picture as health and healing in existence for you.

Healing

As alternative medicine enters deeper into the consciousness of humanity, it opens the door to all sorts of different ways in which a person can find healing. In the part of the *Daily Telegraph* given over to health news recently there was an article about massage and aromatherapy being used in hospitals and nurses being trained to use these techniques to help geriatrics and the terminally ill. Apparently they are also being used to calm and relax pregnant women. The dream is to unite the unconventional with the orthodox so as to bring the benefits of both to the patients.

It has been said with some truth that there is only one sickness and that is *congestion*, that is a block to the flow of life. In the body politic we manage to block the flow of ideas and so progress too is blocked.

People sometimes wonder how colour can cure. It is through the aura that colour therapy operates. Each part of the body is controlled by a different colour. The reason this is so is because each organ has a different rate of vibration, and this is equivalent to a certain colour. If a particular organ is diseased it will have a low rating when tested by the pendulum. Colour therapy introduces the colour needed to correct the imbalance of the organ and it will then be returned to health and the reading will be normal.

Colour healing is a delicate matter, for you are treating the whole person, not just a symptom. You have to look to the weakest link in order to restore the body to health.

Consider indigo blue. It is often used where there is

some congestion of the lungs, and it also stops ulceration and inflammation. Each colour has a different application and meaning.

Colour healing can also be used for patients with mental diseases. In Worcester, Mass., USA, the state hospital for mental patients has set up a wonderful room known as the 'green room'. This is like a cavern at the bottom of the sea — the walls are light green, there are green shades at the windows and the sunlight filters through them producing a green light in the room. There are four large bathtubs, also green, and the whole atmosphere is described as one of complete tranquillity. A wonderful therapy for agitated patients.

Here the doctors have found that light green beds in the ward also help to calm disturbed patients, especially if this is coupled with pale green, grey or yellow walls. This gives a more cheery atmosphere and makes it all more home-like.

As we have mentioned before, scarlet and orange are exciting and stimulating. Yellow is mentally stimulating and green is a neutral and a building colour, while violet and purple are subduing. Therefore, if a patient is melancholy or depressed, he is to be placed in a stimulating atmosphere, and if he is excited he needs calming colours.

Red is such a warm, aggressive colour, it needs to be used with discretion. Red and yellow combined in a room are cheering. Blue is a cooling colour and can be depressing for some people, but it is a good antidote to high blood pressure. Grey is a neutral colour and creates a happy atmosphere between cheerfulness and gloom.

Man's Seven Subtle Bodies

Esoteric science gives a man a sevenfold nature of subtle bodies and the aura is the expression of that nature. The teaching is that man has not only a physical body, but that he has, so to speak, a foot on other planes of being beyond the physical. Few will dispute that man has an intellectual and an emotional nature and so can, in common with his fellow human beings, operate on these planes as well as through his physical body.

The seven aspects of man are not separate states distinct from one another, but are currents of thought and feeling within the whole ocean of consciousness, and often overlap. Man then is a more complex creature than orthodox science allows or knows, for potentially he has these seven aspects which make up his complete being, but of course many people at present experience very little development on the higher vehicles.

The sevenfold division of man's nature is usually classified in the following levels of consciousness:

1. Physical Etheric Plane
2. Astral Plane
3. Lower Mental Plane
4. Higher Mental Plane
5. Spiritual Causal Plane
6. Intuitional Plane
7. Divine or Absolute Plane

To the skilled clairvoyant, or one who uses the Kilner screen, the aura will reveal a man's character, his emotional and mental nature, his state of health and his spiritual development.

Man being — as the Ancient Wisdom has always contended — a septenary being, the auric emanation consists of seven distinct units or waves of light, encircling the subject in an oval-shaped conformation. The extent and strength of the aura varies considerably from person to person, depending on the state of health, mental and emotional state, and evolutionary status.

The *first* aura is the one emanating from the physical etheric body and it is this cloud-shaped formation that most people see first when they practise seeing the aura. Its base is the centre of the spine. The etheric body, the vital counterpart of the physical, is important as it draws in the *prana* or life energy from the atmosphere and distributes it through the system. In a healthy body, the first aura radiates outwards in straight regular lines from the body's centre. In disease these lines are seen to droop, rather like bent lightning conductors.

The *second* aura emanates from the astral, or the emotional centre in the spleen, and encircles the astral body, extending about 12 to 18 inches from the body. Every change of thought or emotion causes a change in this aura. It vibrates and changes continually. In harmony, it should be bright and luminous, showing emotional balance.

The *third* aura is the expression of man's intellectual make-up and its strength depends upon the development of his faculties, which in turn partly depends upon the education he has enjoyed. It is oval, emitting a radiant pale yellow colour as it develops. In the intelligent, well-balanced person, the aura is bright and shiny, but where the mind is depraved there are dark spots which dull its brightness.

The *fourth* aura is the emanation of man's higher mind or soul principle. Its colour tone is green. Here we have the realm of imagination, inspiration and intuition, of creativity in art and literature.

The *fifth* aura interpenetrates the foregoing auras. This aura manifests the essence of spirit in man. Occult science teaches us that conditions in the lower forms of consciousness are the result of forces within the spiritual body. It is the receiving station for all the doings of the lower aspects and records the impressions received by them. The fifth aura is most important, for it is the point of union between the cosmos and the individual. There exists a delicate band between the individual life and the ocean of consciousness shared by all.

The *sixth* and *seventh* auras are higher ones belonging

rather to cosmic aspects than to individuals in particular. The average man has just not developed that far, and these auras would only be seen around the bodies of initiates and masters.

Chakras (Power Centres)

So we all have seven subtle bodies or levels of consciousness, ranging from the grossest, the physical, to the most spiritual or finest. These seven bodies all interpenetrate and are joined to the physical at the seven power centres or *chakras* in the spine. Through these centres and the rays which they attract, we are in touch with, and affected by, all the seven planes of consciousness. Each chakra attracts to itself a predominant colour ray which is necessary to the harmony of the whole individual.

A condition of disharmony implies that either too much or too little of a particular colour vibration is present. This may occur through some agency affecting us from outside, such as an accident or epidemic, or inwardly through the mind entertaining too many negative thoughts and so changing the vibrations in this way.

A small boy, upon being asked how he would describe God, said simply, 'I think of Him as Light.' Looked at from the angle of colour and its place in our lives, this is a very apt description, for all life is energy vibrating at a different rate. Each vibration has a corresponding colour and all colour rays emanate from the central source, the *Great White Light* or *Logos*, as we are instructed by the Ancient Teachings. In fact, as with everything else in life, there is an outer form to be perceived by our senses and an inner or hidden meaning to be discovered. So we come to discuss the chakras, through which the primal energy in the shape of white light, is drawn into the body through the power centres. Each chakra absorbs a special current of vital energy through its particular colour ray from the physical environment and from higher levels of consciousness.

In the completely healthy body the energy flows in harmoniously, and is absorbed through the chakras. The opposite occurs, however, where there is a blockage of one kind or another in one of the bodies.

If the cosmic energy stopped at the fourth level, say, then there would be some distortion in the way of thinking and this distortion would be transmitted to the astral and the physical/etheric bodies and so be experienced as some form of illness or dis-harmony in the physical body. The higher bodies affect the lower, but not vice versa.

The Seven Primary Rays

Centres which predominantly attract these rays

1. Red   The lowest centre in the base of the spine.
2. Orange   In the small of the back, to the left-hand side of the spine. (Splenic centre.)
3. Yellow   Middle of the back over the kidneys. (Solar plexus centre.)
4. Green   Between the shoulder blades in line with the heart.
5. Blue   At the base of the skull. (Throat centre.)
6. Indigo   In the forehead, the pineal gland. (Brow centre)
7. Violet   In the dome of the head. (Pituitary centre.)

There are seven main chakras, each under a particular colour. These are seen clairvoyantly as continually moving, great wheel-like vortices situated in the etheric body — the pattern on which the physical is built. These chakras or vortices link with the spine at definite intervals.

Light is a force stimulating to growth; every living thing depends upon it to build and maintain its form. Light, therefore, whose source is solar energy, is one of the greatest healing forces. In the human being energy is drawn in through the chakras and distributed over the whole body. The chakras draw in their own specialized colours, as listed above, so that the two lowest centres, the *red* and *orange*, draw in energy from the sunlight and this energy is directed through the body.

The *red* and the *orange chakras* govern the physical and etheric level in man and supply the vital energies needed by these bodies, although it should be mentioned that the activity of the chakras is not localized but interpenetrative. The *yellow chakra* governs the lower mental level, but also has to do with emotional influences. The *green chakra*, called the heart centre, governs the higher mind but also influences the higher emotions such as sympathy, kindness, understanding and compassion. The *blue* or *throat chakra* is the centre of religious and spiritual instincts. The *blue*, *red* and *yellow chakras* need to work in harmony for there to be genuine health of mind and body.

The *indigo* and *violet chakras* are both transcendental and rule the higher aspirations of the soul. These can express clairvoyance, spiritual intuition, or healing.

Colour healing can thus restore the balance where disease has caused a *blocking* or slowing down of the energy intake through the chakras or its circulation.

Diagnosis is made by clairvoyance, or by the use of aids to make the aura visible to those without psychic vision. The discoloured area showing disease can be treated by rays to clear the blockages. Colour breathing can also be advocated to hasten recovery or simply to maintain good health. Clairvoyant vision shows that where the aura is ragged or droopy and colour breathing is practised, there is an immediate revival of the frayed aura with the new intake of vitality.

Just as each major colour has seven intrinsic elements in its composition, so in each colour one of the seven elements predominates (see the following table). For instance, in number one a physical element predominates;

this is the lowest centre at the base of the spine. In number five a specific healing element predominates; this is the throat centre and its colour is *blue*.

Base centre.	1.	A physical element.
Splenic centre.	2.	A vitality element.
Solar plexus centre.	3.	A psychological element.
Heart centre.	4.	A harmonizing element.
Throat centre.	5.	A specific healing element.
Brow centre.	6.	An element of inspiration and intuition.
Pituitary centre.	7.	A spiritual element.

A Spiritual Force

Colour healing is not only a physical but a spiritual force, and so forms a link between our physical bodies and the finer forces or vibrations of higher levels of consciousness and spiritual growth. The use is not confined to spiritual or unorthodox healers, it is also used by orthodox practitioners, although perhaps the latter tend to use the more dangerous — because more powerful — infra-red and ultra-violet rays. However, it is possible that colour healing could also be the link or bridge between the orthodox and unorthodox disciplines, so that in the end the old orthodox idea of treating the physical body alone may die the death and new ideas, taking into account the wholeness of man and his entire *force field*, may benefit humanity mightily. It has many advantages over other methods of healing, being harmless and able to reach the subtle bodies, where all disease starts. Furthermore it makes possible early diagnosis through auric examination long before the disease manifests in the physical body, and it cannot cause side effects.

CHAPTER THREE

THE SEVEN MAJOR RAYS

As explained in the previous chapter, cosmic energy in the shape of light rays is drawn into the body through the chakras or power centres, distributed along the spine, and flows through the body, vitalizing it. Where there are blockages for whatever reason, this impoverishes the body and disease sets in.

The theory on which colour healing is based is that everyone is individual in their requirements of specific colours and that health of mind and body is based upon the body obtaining a balanced flow according to these requirements, that is, sufficient to enable the body to rebuild, restore and revitalize every organ in order to maintain its health and freedom from disease.

Just as man has seven bodies or levels of consciousness, so there are seven chakras and seven major rays.

The Red Cosmic Ray

This is the ray which supplies our physical bodies with energy and vitality. It is drawn in through the *base chakra* at the root of the spine and correlates with the *coccygeal* or *gonad centre*. The physical vitality of the body depends upon the correct and sufficient intake of the *red* ray, particularly so far as the creative, procreative and restorative functions are concerned.

Treatment with the *red* ray stimulates this centre. It promotes heat and body temperature, stimulates the circulation of the blood and gets the adrenalin going. It disperses feelings of tiredness and inertia, as well as chronic chills or colds; its action is always expansive. Diet to help the action of *red* rays should include beetroot, radishes, black cherries, damsons, plums, spinach, cresses and currants — in fact any vegetables and fruits containing iron. Healers also often suggest that the patient drink several tumblerfuls of *red* ray-charged water. This is water that has absorbed the *red* rays from the sun being filtered through a red screen. The effect of the *red* ray, psychologically and on the nervous system, is always uplifting, giving more confidence, initiative, overcoming depression and inertia, stimulating will-power and courage.

The use of the *red* ray could be indicated in cases of anaemia, paralysis, poor circulation, and disorders of the blood where the vitality is depleted or the mental state is one of depression, fear or worry.

The Orange Cosmic Ray

The *orange* ray controls the *second chakra*, the *splenic centre*, and it assists in the assimilative, distributory and circulatory processes of the body. It has a powerful tonic effect, frees the bodily and mental functions, gives both physical energy and mental stimulation. It has often been called the *wisdom ray*. Lying as it does midway between the physical *red* ray, and the mental *yellow* ray, it has an action on both the physical vitality and the intellect. Diet to help the action of *orange* rays includes most orange-skinned vegetables and fruits — oranges, tangerines, apricots, mangoes, peaches, cantaloup melons, carrots and swedes — and also a glass or two of orange-charged water.

Both the *orange* and *red* rays are powerful and treatment should never be used indiscriminately. Each patient is unique and must be treated as such.

Psychologically, the *orange* ray is wonderful for removing repressions and inhibitions, it helps to broaden the mind and to open it to new ideas, and where there is mental retardation it is a great help in raising the mental level. As it broadens the mind, it brings more understanding and tolerance. Like the *red* ray it also supplies courage and the power to cope with life.

As the *orange* ray is absorbed through the *splenic centre*, so it can be used for the treatment of disorders and infections of the spleen, also for kidney diseases. Bronchitis and other chest troubles can be treated with the *orange* ray. Gallstones respond to treatment by the *orange* ray, as does paralysis of any emotional origin.

The Yellow Cosmic Ray

Next to white, this is the ray giving out the maximum light. It is absorbed through the *third chakra*, or the *solar plexus*, which is really a very important centre for the whole nervous system and it controls the digestive processes as well. Its action is eliminative on the liver and intestines so that it is a purifier for the whole system, but particularly for the skin, where it has powerful healing properties. It is a *mental ray*, and stimulates the intellectual faculties. Diet to help the action of the *yellow* ray consists basically of yellow-skinned vegetables and fruit such as lemons, bananas, grapefruit, pineapples and sweetcorn. Again, many healers charge water in sunlight through a yellow filter and prescribe it for their patients.

Psychologically, the *yellow* ray stimulates the logical mind and the reasoning powers. It also aids self-control through inspiring the higher faculties. We are stimulated and our spirits raised merely by looking at yellow and orange, for these colours resemble most closely the lovely golden sunshine which our bodies crave. So yellow is a colour which brings a harmonious attitude to life, providing balance and optimism.

The use of the *yellow* ray could be indicated in cases of nervous exhaustion, where there are skin troubles, indigestion and the related complaints of constipation, liver trouble and diabetes.

The Green Cosmic Ray

Green is the colour of nature, of balance, peace and harmony. When we who live in the towns seek refreshment and contentment, we drive out into the country, even if this can only be for a few hours on Sundays! Instinctively we know that the green of the countryside will be restorative and soothing. It is the *midway* mark in the colour spectrum between the heat end of the spectrum and the electric end.

This is the ray which is absorbed by the *heart chakra* and controls the *cardiac centre*. Green is a mixture of blue and yellow, and strongly influences the heart and blood pressure. In fact chlorophyll, which is produced by plants, can now be chemically synthesized, and is produced and marketed for sustaining the heart action. It also has a wonderful soothing effect upon the nerves and probably it is its lack in some of the built-up areas and concrete jungles designed by modern architects that accounts for the rising waves of crime and delinquency. Diet to help the action of the *green* ray is the use of all green vegetables and fruits that are neither acidulous nor alkaline in reaction.

Psychologically the *green* ray brings a feeling of renewal, of new life, freshness and brightness, rather like the coming of spring. This is the ray which governs not only the *physical* heart, but also emotional problems and repressions which bring on heart attacks. These are often due to a fear of giving, a fear of involvement or of being hurt; if such emotional and psychological problems continue over a long period they can all too easily end up in high blood pressure and heart attacks.

Therefore, the *green* ray, experienced by getting away from it all into the country or at least into your garden, is a wonderful 'builder-upper' and restorer for the heart, and also for blood pressure and ulcers. It can also be used for alleviating headaches and 'flu. As cancer is an imbalance of the cells, so *green*, the harmonizer and balancer, can be used to neutralize the extreme disharmony of malignant cells, restore harmony to the nervous system and tune up the whole body.

The Blue Cosmic Ray

Just as the *red* ray is an expander and stimulator, so the *blue* ray is the opposite, so far as the previous group of *red/orange/yellow* rays are concerned, for it is the contractor and restrictor. It is the 'steadier-upper' and slows things down so that it can combat infectious diseases where there is a rise in temperature. Its great property is that of an antiseptic; its light is cooling and astringent. *Blue* is the colour of the throat centre — the centre which controls man's greatest power of self-expression, speech. Diet to help the action of the *blue* ray consists of all blue fruits and vegetables such as grapes, blackberries (which are often a deep blue), blue plums, bilberries, and the taking of a glass or so of blue-charged water every day.

Psychologically, the *blue* ray can bring quiet and peace

of mind, particularly where there has been an over-excited state, such as one bordering on hysteria. It can in fact be so relaxing that the common saying, 'I feel blue', would imply too much blue and the need for a little 'zip up and go' *red* or *orange*.

The *blue* ray can be used to alleviate many diverse ailments such as throat troubles of all kinds, fevers and children's ailments, such as measles and mumps, many inflammations, spasms, stings, itchings and headaches. It is also useful for shock, insomnia and period pains.

The Indigo Cosmic Ray

The *indigo* ray is drawn in and circulated by the chakra behind the brow, often called the *third eye*. It is said to control the *pineal gland*, and is a wonderful purifier of the blood stream. Like the *orange* ray, it helps to broaden the mind and free it of fears and inhibitions. *Indigo* is a combination of deep blue and a small amount of steadying red.

The pineal gland has to do with the nervous, mental and psychic potential of a man, so that the organs of sight and hearing are under the influence of the *indigo* ray. It is probably for this reason that the *indigo* ray is a powerful anaesthetic — using the *indigo* ray is a very safe way of gaining anaesthesia, for consciousness is maintained but there is complete insensitivity to pain. Diet to help the action of the *indigo* ray can include the foods listed under the *blue* ray and those which will be given for the *violet* ray too.

Psychologically, it clears and cleans the psychic currents of the body, even having a powerful effect on serious mental complaints such as obsession and other forms of psychosis. The *indigo* ray is purifying and stabilizing in cases where fears and repressions have produced a serious mental complaint.

In treatment the *indigo* ray can be used to treat any diseases of the eyes, ears and nose, also diseases of the lungs, asthma and dyspepsia. Deafness can sometimes be the result of a refusal to hear the voice of conscience or enlightenment, or merely the words of those close to the patient. Instead there is an in-turning of attention. Naturally, this is not always so, but in any case the *indigo* ray can be of great help in any ear, nose, or throat problem.

The Violet Cosmic Ray

This has the highest vibration of all the cosmic energy rays. It controls the *crown chakra* in the head, and is linked with the *pituitary gland*, which is a centre of intuitive and spiritual understanding. The *violet* ray acts in a most soothing and tranquillizing manner upon frayed nervous systems, of which there are plenty today. However, its usefulness in terms of response is mainly for those who are nervous and highly-strung by nature. Artists, actors and musicians often suffer from personality disorders and it is the violet ray which can restore them to peace and calm.

The diet to be used together with charged waters consists of such foods as recommended for the *indigo* ray, and aubergines, purple grapes, blackberries, purple broccoli and beetroot.

Psychologically, this is the *ray de luxe*, which has a wonderful healing effect on all forms of neurosis and neurotic manifestations. It can be used to assist the development of the spiritual, intuitive faculty. Before beginning meditation or concentration exercises, the colour could be visualized or else a small cloth of that colour could be placed on a table in front of you as an aid to stimulating the psychic and spiritual faculties.

In treatment *violet* can be used for all mental and nervous disease, also for rheumatism, concussion, tumours, cerebro-spinal meningitis, kidney and bladder diseases.

The Ancient Wisdom teaches that colour names and the numbers of each chakra and ray are symbols for great forces which emanate from the Supreme Power behind all manifestation. Each of the seven rays stands for one of the great evolutionary periods through which humanity has to pass. Everything in existence is dependent upon these great cosmic radiations, not only this earth, but all the other planes of manifestation, the etheric, astral, mental and spiritual planes which make up the universe, all are dependent on this same cosmic power of Light.

The seven rays represent stages in evolutionary progress. The first three rays, the *red*, *orange* and *yellow*, have already passed and humanity is now in the evolutionary period of the *green* ray, the mid-point and the lowest point of immersion in matter. Ahead the outlook is brighter, a period of progress awaits humanity, with an advance into the higher, more harmonious *blue* ray and so to the finer conditions of the *indigo* and *violet* rays.

As these rays and their numbers are symbols of great *Forces* with which we are surrounded every day of our lives, so each one of us has command of particular gifts which are part of our own potential for development in terms of material or creative success, and this we will see in a later chapter devoted to music, colour and number in our lives.

Dr Edwin D. Babbit in *The Principles of Light and Colour* (published in 1878), tells us how, after many years of research into colour therapy, he developed the ability with his inner vision to see colours swirling around him in a great ocean of flashing light, and describes the experiences as being beyond belief in glory. Everything became a mass of luminous, swirling radiations flowing into, through, and from, everything. He concluded that there was a basically spiritual force from which *all* healing must come of whatever nature. It is simply the channels we use to effect the healing that differ.

CHAPTER FOUR

DIAGNOSIS AND TREATMENT

When we think about healing we usually consider only the physical body of flesh and muscle that we can see, but it is well to remember that the Ancient Wisdom teaches that this body consists of two parts, one visible and the other invisible or 'subtle'. This latter is the vital body or 'etheric double'. Both are composed of physical matter and both are cast off at death. The etheric body is the source of all physical vitality and the absorber and transmitter of energy through the system. This double is an exact replica of the visible body, its organs corresponding exactly with the physical organism, hence disease begins first in the etheric body, or in one of the higher bodies, before it attacks the physical; there can, therefore, be an early diagnosis of the impending disease.

Two Nervous Systems

Operation of the physical organism depends upon the efficient functioning of the nervous systems, of which there are two. The involuntary system, not under the control of the will, operates all the automatic functions of the body, such as heart beating and breathing, without our having to worry about them; in fact if we did we would probably stop their functioning.

The other nervous system is voluntary and is centred on the brain, spinal cord and solar plexus. Through this system we think, feel and act. If these centres are defective in any way, man's expression in the physical world is imperfect to the extent of the damage.

Colour rays affect the condition of both the etheric and physical cells. The etheric body is the connecting link between the physical senses and the higher forces, and in health the vital or etheric body energizes the physical body. To clairvoyant or trained vision, the aura of the etheric body is visible as a luminous outline of a pale golden colour radiating outwards in every direction. These radiations, when strong and healthy, can get rid of germs and infections through their strength and vitality, but in ill health the etheric strength is depleted, unable to absorb the correct amount of energy, and the radiations — lacking vital force — appear to the clairvoyant as drooping lines.

Colour healing aims to build up the etheric body through applying the correct colour vibrations to the chakras, which then become capable of vitalizing the physical body.

Methods of Diagnosis

There are three main methods of diagnosis: by psychic perception, by the use of the Kilner screen — whereby the conditions on the astral and etheric levels can be ascertained — and by radiesthesia, or the use of ESP functioning through the pendulum.

I am told that practitioners can map the outline of the aura by using certain designs of the pendulum. To the radiesthetist each colour has its own particular vibration and this they can pick up by observing the swing of the pendulum. Allied to this is the diagnostic and treatment instrument; attunement is made through a sample spot of blood, a hair snippet or even a signature. An expert can make a complete health diagnosis and then treat the patient.

The trained psychic is aware of the different levels of consciousness through which man works, his sevenfold potential contained within the one, all with their different radiations making up the aura or the ovoid electro-magnetic field with which we are all surrounded. Here is the outward expression of the man, his physical, emotional, lower and higher, mental and spiritual potentials. To the psychic, the dullness or patchiness of colour will be observable and treatment can be given at the required level. Some psychics are so gifted that they do not even require the presence of the patient, but can diagnose at a distance provided they have an article belonging to the person in their hands.

So far as the third method of diagnosis is concerned, by means of radiesthesia and the radionic instrument, this will be very similar to the psychic investigation and naturally will vary according to the training and experience of the practitioner. Details on the use of the pendulum are given later in this chapter.

The Kilner Screen

Finally we come to the method using the Kilner screen, pioneered by Dr Kilner. He was convinced that it could be a much more effective way of diagnosis, as ill health would show up in the aura before the physical symptoms appeared.

The Kilner screen is composed of two pieces of glass between which has been poured a solution of dicyanin, a dye of indigo-violet colour, which considerably sharpens the vision of the observer. Ideally a special diagnosing cabinet would be built where the patient can be seated, clad only in a black silk robe to facilitate vision. The condition of the lower auras can then be seen. If a special cabinet is not possible, then the diagnostician should seat the patient in a darkened room. After a while the emanations from the etheric body will become visible.

It should be mentioned that in an emergency it is often necessary to diagnose through symptoms, the person's general demeanour, and expressed habits. Remember that there are two principal colours, the heating *red/orange* and the cooling *blue/violet*, with *green* representing the mid-point, the balance or harmonizer.

Broadly the aim of the healer is to find out which of these opposing colours is wanting in the patient and how to cure the complaint. For instance, if the person is inclined to be depressed, is slow in reaction, has no energy or appetite, then he requires the *red/orange* colours rays. If he is impatient, choleric, overactive or has a raised temperature, he requires the *blue/violet* rays to cool him.

Locating the Diseased Organ

There are two main types of healing: contact and absent. In both cases the aim of healing is to restore the vitality to the etheric vehicle through the projection of colour rays; these are then absorbed by the power centres interpenetrating the spine. The decision as to which centre the ray should be directed to will depend upon the position of the diseased organ.

Another method open to those with sensitive finger tips or hands — if psychic vision is not developed — is to pass the right hand over the body until the vibration of the fingers, or in some people the tingling of the palm and a heat sensation, show that the seat of the trouble has been located. This is somewhat similar to the use of the pendulum for diagnosis and either the hand or the pendulum could be used to pick out the colour ray to be used. Naturally a broad sample card of colours well depicted would have to be used for the latter method.

Treatment can be either diffused over the body or concentrated. Continuity of treatment is important and most healers seem to agree that treatment should last for about 25 to 30 minutes. Overall treatment consists in focusing the lamps — or in some cases the hands — to direct the colour, through thought-power, over the whole body, but especially over the back. The patient either lies or sits in a relaxed position, with the upper half of the body uncovered. This is a wonderful tonic for revitalizing and toning up the body.

Coloured Filters

In concentrated treatment the colour lamp with the appropriate filter for the particular disharmony is focused on the affected area only. This treatment usually lasts about 15 minutes and can be followed by the general overall one. Most healers use a lamp or projector into which different coloured filters can be inserted. A more elaborate electrical colour treatment apparatus is an electro-thermolume cabinet. The patient sits in the cabinet and is bathed in colour from colour screens fixed at the front of the cabinet.

Another often used and effective method is through the use of colour-solarized water. Dr Babbitt suggests that not only can water be charged, but also milk, sugar and pulverized gum arabic, as these substances are fairly neutral and so can be used to take any colour charge required. The method is either to place the water in a jar or a glass of the required colour and leave it out in sunlight for an hour or two, or to place coloured paper over the glass or jar, again of course of the required colour. The patient then drinks the solarized water.

Colour Breathing and Visualization

Visualization is now being used quite extensively in psychotherapy, whether in groups or in individual work. It can also be used by the colour therapist and by the lay person wishing to treat him or herself. It is possible to use colour breathing and visualization for youth and beauty as well as for health.

Of course many people will not believe the effect colour has on the human body and psyche. However the reports of scientists and doctors who have studied colour and done extensive research on it will prove an eye-opener to the sceptics. Colour is an energy, a wavelength just as the other different forms which produce the telephone, radio, TV, radar, laser beams and other miracles of modern technology. Colour has wavelengths which can affect living tissue. Humans are now receiving quite a few mixed vibrations from our TV sets, and I warrant it will not be long before someone gets on to querying how good it is for the human body to be exposed for so many hours a day to the particular wavelengths continually being emitted by television.

We mentioned earlier that man has seven subtle bodies, which are invisible to usual sight, interpenetrate and are joined to the physical at the seven power centres or chakras in the spine. In visualization and breathing colour we are only concerned with one level of consciousness above the physical and that is the etheric, which is an exact duplicate of the physical body, but vibrates at a much higher, lighter rate than the grosser, denser, physical body. It is the pattern upon which the physical was originally built. Research has shown, as stated earlier, that disease often registers in the etheric body before it actually appears in the physical and can be seen to clairvoyant sight as a discolouration in the aura at the disease point. The theory then developed by some colour therapists is that you can influence your own physical body, either for health or appearance, through the etheric body. This theory is set out clearly by Roland T. Hunt, Ivah Berg Whitten and Linda Clark and Yvonne Martine, who did both practical work and research in this field with much success.

Esoteric teaching has always been that thoughts are things and that continual bright and cheerful thoughts keep the physical body in good health. The opposite is true of pessimistic and depressing thoughts or even ones where the emotions are stirred up and chaotic. This affects the physical body adversely, so it is said. It is the continual holding of negative thoughts and attitudes which eventually is said to result in physical weakness.

We can as easily present positive, happy, forward-looking thoughts to the etheric body as we can a depressing mélange of fear and anticipation. We must visualize what we want, *not* what we don't want! It is this powerful visualization of what we do want that will project this to the etheric body. Continuity and persistence are necessary for success, no use thinking, 'Well, I'll just try this out tonight, I expect to see results tomorrow.' Generally, many tomorrows must take place before you will get a satisfactory result. After all, you are working to change something in yourself either physically or psychologically. The hardest things to change, as you may have noticed, are people's attitudes and habits, often spanning a lifetime — or even more than one if you are a believer in life after life, a reincarnationist.

So to be successful we must be patient and persistent.

We must not only visualize what we want and be able to hold the picture clearly in our minds, but we must also *think* of what we want. Powerful thinking is what is needed, nothing half-hearted will do. One could compare the etheric to a computer, which of course has to be programmed to produce anything at all. So your blueprint for the new 'you' in some respect must be positive and you must not neglect to look after your nutrition and see that you give the body those things which it needs to grow and stay beautiful and healthy.

To get good results, whatever you wish to improve or change in yourself, you must be prepared to work seriously at it, to do it regularly and to perfect your techniques of visualization and breathing. Do add colour to perfect your work.

Beauty Colour Breathing

The very first 'must' is relaxation, both of mind and body — a sort of detached meditative state. This of course applies whatever type of work we wish to do along inner lines of endeavour.

Linda Clark and Yvonne Martine suggest we breathe in pink air at eye level for several breaths. Then breathe in the pink air and mentally direct it to the area you wish to improve as follows:

1. While holding your breath visualize the area as perfect.
2. Do this three times.
3. Offer your thanks for help.
4. If necessary repeat for other areas.
5. Put the whole thing out of your mind until your next session.

This is best done on waking and on going to sleep.

Colour Breathing for Health

Although Linda Clark and Yvonne Martine are forbidden under US laws from publishing any health claims for colour breathing, they can state where they have benefited themselves and suggest that there are no side effects and you have nothing to lose in trying out the suggestions. In their book, *Health, Youth and Beauty Through Colour Breathing* (Celestial Arts, US, 1976), Yvonne tells of how some years back she had had a series of light heart attacks, was suffering from arthritis, was 20 pounds underweight and was thoroughly worn out and exhausted. Her doctor had given her five years to live. She says, 'Using colour breathing cleared my arthritis in one month. All the knobs in my body disappeared after using turquoise colour breathing for that length of time. All this success was later confirmed by my doctor, who did not know how I had become well again. Surprisingly, the liver spots I had on my hands and face took four years to disappear. My weight also became normal and I am in perfect health today.'

Yvonne also had the misfortune to break her leg, but was able to heal it far quicker than would have been possible by orthodox methods. She was able to discard the cast after only three weeks. After this, continuation of the colour breathing and visualization returned the limb to perfect health.

It seems true to say that most people die from the accumulation of toxins in the body. The late Roland Hunt, the internationally-known colour expert, concentrated on one colour for cleansing congestion in each area and organ of the body. He named this cleansing process *clarification*, and the single cleansing colour the *light of clarification*, which is a deep violet or medium purple, about the shade of Parma violets.

He stated that the persistent beaming of this colour on various parts of the body dissolved congestion from a solid to a fluid state and that within 24 hours after the clarification there might well be a feeling of discomfort while the toxins were being discharged from the body. This might include sinus discharge, kidney or intestinal activity. He felt that nerves, circulation and other unresolved pressures of many kinds benefited from the cleansing process.

Here is Roland Hunt's method. Beginning at the top of the head and holding his palms facing downward toward the crown of the head, he would visualize a beam of this deep violet light focusing on the glands of the head, the pineal and the pituitary. He suggested holding his palms about nine inches away from the area to be treated. If there was some congestion in the area the resistance would be noted in the palms, which would feel warm. Once the resistance was dissolved the palms would feel cool, showing it was time to move on to the next area. Yvonne Martine notes that when she used this treatment, it worked best for her at three and not nine inches away from the body. She also noticed that it was the area treated and not the palms of her hands which heated up. Which I think only goes to show that there are always individual reactions and individual ways of using healing techniques.

After finishing the crown of the head, Hunt's continuing instruction for clearing the toxins was to place the left hand in front of the brow and the right hand directly behind it at the back of the head. He would then move his left hand to the bridge of the nose and his right hand to the base of the brain.

The next position was putting each hand at the level of the ears and the parotid glands. Ear discharge might result.

The next placement was on the sides of the neck, below the ear, over the carotid and lymph glands for emotional and blood pressure balance.

Next Hunt would place his left hand over the thyroid and parathyroid (in the front of the neck) and the right hand over the *occiput* at the back of the neck where the head joins the neck. Then he placed both hands fairly close together over the lungs, then the right hand over the thymus, then the heart. Then he lowered his hands over the digestive organs, the liver, gall bladder, pancreas and spleen, later over the intestines and colon. Finally, reaching behind him, he placed one hand over each kidney, in the small of the back, and the adrenals which lie atop of each kidney.

Roland Hunt stated that this session might take as long as 40 minutes and should not be done more frequently than once than every other day.

Yvonne Martine has her own method for cleansing and healing an area. She breathes as for the beauty routine, but merely uses different colours. First if an area of the body is causing trouble she floods it with a pinkish orange, a soft, apricot orange. Then on the holding breath, after inhaling the colour, she holds the orange where it is needed if there is pain, as in the case of a fracture, or, if no pain is present, merely to wake up the cells to activate them. After this she applies a deep violet to cleanse the cells in the disturbed area. She follows this with the colour needed for the healing of the particular condition. Yvonne uses this method three times a day — upon waking, at midday and upon retiring.

There has always been a yogic method of healing, probably several. In the method described here, the therapist focuses the necessary colour on the area to be healed, breathing through her nose, with her mouth closed. She inhales slowly and rhythmically to the count of five, holds the breath to the count of ten, during which time she visualizes the area needing healing as perfect; then exhales to the count of five. She repeats this cycle five times, giving thanks at the end *knowing* that the healing is being done. This series of five cycles should be done only once daily. It is said that this method stimulates the 72,000 *Nadis*, or acupuncture points, in the body.

At this point it might be helpful to describe what is

known in yoga as the complete breath. This is done by inhaling, during which time the stomach balloons outward. While holding this outward position, I mentally visualize the breath going upward to the lungs, completely filling them. If you are going to use this breath for treating, as the yogis do, you do it at this point. Then, as you exhale, pull your stomach in. To check yourself and see if you are doing the breath properly, you put one hand on your stomach or lower abdomen, and the other on your lungs. As you inhale, the hand on the stomach should rise as the stomach distends. The hand on the lungs remains quiet, since the air expands the lungs internally and sideways without rising upwards. When you exhale, the hand on your abdomen goes inward with it. Later, you can direct the breath elsewhere in your body.

Regarding the colours to use on any particular area, it seems that many people use gold to heal everywhere and it is the experience of many workers in this field that if another colour is required that colour will make its appearance although you may have started with gold.

One colour therapist noted an interesting experience. She had begun to suffer hair loss, so every morning during her meditation she used the complete breath (which she mentally coloured golden as used by others for general healing purposes) and she carried it mentally from her lungs upward to the scalp and affirmed either audibly or silently, 'This healing breath is now stimulating a thick growth of hair on my head.' She held it there for a short while, and repeated this breath three times. To her astonishment, somewhere along the way between the second and third breath, her head became very warm. Something was obviously happening and she gave thanks, remembering that circulation follows attention.

Later at the same session she used the pink breath for beautiful, thick hair, then turned her mind off the whole subject.

Several weeks later, she discovered a short bristling

stubble forming on her scalp at the base of the longer hairs. That growth continued to an inch in length and a new second bristle began. She was on her way to the thick, beautiful hair she had wanted. She also gives a tip to hold concentration, which is essential to success in this particular field. She tells us to visualize the golden healing colour as coming from a spotlight held in the hand above the problem area.

Yvonne Martine uses the following colours in her work with colour healing for various conditions:

Pink Breath: For wrinkles, acne, sagginess, puffiness, crepiness and looseness of the skin anywhere on face or body.

Turquoise Breath: Blue-green has created changes in the circulatory system, relieved respiratory ailments, arthritis, some heart and gastric conditions, removed excess fat when alternated with pink and is also used to increase weight. Yvonne Martine says to use turquoise three times, then pink three times, but visualize the desired outline of the body in pink. The turquoise is used internally, the pink externally.

Orange: A soft apricot-orange containing some pink removes pain, but does not cure it.

Dark Blue: Dark blue tinged with green, or green with a blue tinge accompanied by an opaque film is used for mending bones.

Sky Blue: This colour has improved memory, intellectual or artistic talents, and can be used for a feeling of relaxation or well-being.

Dark Green: To purify the blood and for any associated diseases.

Grass Green: For success, monetary gain and acquisition of possessions, providing it is qualified with statements such as 'according to God's will'. This must not be used for something illegal or which belongs to someone else. There is enough for all. Yvonne advises spending at least five minutes morning and night seeing yourself surrounded with this colour, and emotionally experience the desired result of what you wish or need.

Pale Green: This has improved vision, and is of benefit for eye injuries or diseases, unless involved with the circulation, nerves, etc, in which case the desired colour for these conditions should be used. According to Yvonne, send the pale green to the solar plexus first then to the eyes. Repeat three times; give thanks.

Medium Green: This colour can be used to alter bad habits and so change the personality for the better. Yvonne advised breathing in the medium green, sending it first to the solar plexus, then transferring to the heart and head areas at least three times in each area. Visualize the new personality as you wish to be. This will require six breaths at each session.

Purple Breath: This can be used for both physical and emotional disturbances. If dangerous conditions are present Yvonne suggests you visualize the purple breath rising up from the feet and enveloping the whole body, while asking that any danger or disturbance be eliminated according to God's will. Then immediately follow this by visualizing a white light or cocoon to insulate you and continue to give you protection.

Pale Orchid: This can be used for spiritual attunement.

Deep Pinkish Rose: For creating a loving rapport with others and has at times also been used for regeneration or organs.

Gold: A general overall healing colour to irradiate you from head to toe. This colour can often be used when in doubt as to what to use.

Lavender or Blue: Very good colours to use for sleeplessness.

These are colours which Yvonne Martine has found to be good, but she does say that often it is best to work out your own method.

On this principle it may be best to use the pendulum to

find out the correct colour to use for any given condition for those of you who are acquainted with its use. In general the pendulum responses are limited to 'yes' and 'no' unless you are a practised radiesthetist in which case you will be able to gain more information.

Mrs Ivah Berg Whitten, of whom we have spoken earlier, was a lecturer and teacher of colour breathing, and she was also a highly spiritual person stating that her teachings came from the Masters. She considered it was possible to see the type of thinking which had generally engrossed a person by the condition of the skin. Wrinkles, she says, are the clogging of the pores of the skin with impurities which can be reversed by colour breathing from the feet upwards and flowing outwards at the head into a fountain of colour.

Mrs Whitten also said that everyone has their own soul colour, and finding and using this colour could be the key to success. It may be then that this soul colour can be found by the use of the pendulum.

There are three other colours of importance: the *colour of inspiration*, *colour of activity* and *colour of rest*. Mrs Whitten advises surrounding yourself with your colour of inspiration during meditation (your telephone number to your Higher Self), and when you are weary, she suggests surrounding yourself with your colour of rest. When you are working, then you should surround yourself with your colour of activity.

Now, you can find all these colours once you have trained yourself to use the pendulum — something which may be very quick and easy with some people, while others, even those very gifted, often need a long period of testing and training to get as near to 100 per cent accuracy as possible. If you do not have a pendulum you can buy them quite cheaply at a shop which sells books on alternative medicine and the occult or you can make one by tying a six to eight inch thread on to largish bead on one end and a smaller bead on the other end so the thread won't slip from your fingers. If you are right-handed hold the pendulum in your right hand. If you are left-handed use your left. You may like to rest your elbow on the table while you use the pendulum but you do not have to do so.

Always ask your Higher Self if you may make an enquiry on a subject and if you receive an affirmative then you can proceed. The convention generally used is that the affirmative is for the pendulum to move clockwise of its own accord. If the answer is negative then the pendulum will move anti-clockwise. If it does not move at all then you have not yet made contact with the correct source of guidance. If it moves from side to side then you have not asked the right question and need to rephrase it. *It is very important to have your mind a complete blank as you ask a question.* If you do not do this it is possible for your mind to influence the answer and you will get an answer biased your way.

You *must* remain neutral when you are working with a pendulum. You should also make sure you are not in a direct line with any electrical instrument such as a television. Do not get upset if you do not gain results immediately. Everything takes time to learn and some experience to gain proficiency — the use of the pendulum is no different from anything else.

If no answer comes at first put the pendulum in its box and wait for another time. It is better to keep your pendulum for your sole use. As you become more used to using it it will respond more efficiently.

Just remember always to ask if you may ask this particular question or not before you begin. Do not cheat. If your answers are later proved to be incorrect, you need to improve your technique, own up to the fact that you've a lot to learn and keep trying.

Mrs Whitten said that your soul colour would be one of seven, each one related to the notes in the musical scale.

1. Red   —   musical note C.
2. Orange —   musical note D.

3. Yellow — musical note E.
4. Green — musical note F.
5. Blue — musical note G.
6. Indigo — musical note A.
7. Violet — musical note B.

If your soul colour turns out to be one of the first four on the list of seven, you should recuperate more quickly from illness or overstrain by visualizing and drawing up the colour from the earth's surface, through the soles of your feet, up the base of your spine and upward to the head.

If your soul colour turns out to be one of the last three, you should draw the energy from above, downwards through your head, body and eventually to your feet.

Remember you know you have made contact when the area you are treating warms, for then you know the energy has arrived to do its work and it will then only be a question of time before you achieve your goal.

Your final step in the healing will be an overall visualization on the holding breath and a statement, silently or aloud, that 'I am now radiantly healthy, youthful and beautiful/handsome ' (the latter if you are a man).

How we think and how we feel about our fellow man will be reflected in our face, in the texture of our skin, in our attitudes and in the way we walk and hold ourselves. Everything about ourselves is a giveaway which is unconsciously picked up by others. Their conclusions about us are drawn on these impressions.

I think that learning colour healing and colour breathing is not easy and requires enthusiasm, zest for research and persistence. Also you need to have something of the spirit of the pioneer in your soul, as this is an area of human life which has not been very much researched, certainly not by established medical centres. Like many other fields in alternative medicine it could do with a laboratory dedicated just to finding out something which was known to generations long gone, but which we have lost and have got to find again, for colour healing has wonderful potential, no side effects and no cutting one about with a knife with all the dangers inherent in such practices.

CHAPTER FIVE

COLOURS FOR COMMON DISEASES

Diagnosis, by various methods, is directed at the etheric body and its seven major force centres. The condition and activity of these centres must first of all be assessed, for it is the force fields or the invisible bodies of man, and in particular the etheric, which form the framework or mesh on which the physical vehicle is built, and these determine the vitality activity and health of that body.

The therapist is well aware that correct breathing and adequate fresh air is necessary for health, and he will perhaps suggest exercises of colour breathing to supply the lacks he has diagnosed. He will also remind his patient of the value of sunlight, sea air and the countryside in building up vitality. Nor will he forget the part which vitamins play in supplying the necessary energy to the vital body. This becomes even more important as our food becomes more and more devitalized with additives and preservatives.

The Ancient Wisdom teachings identify seven major chakras along the spine and in the head. These are wheels of rotating subtle matter and represent energy centres. The organs of the body have affinity with each of these. The *red chakra* at the base of the spine controls the functioning of the *creative and reproductive system*. This is the focus for the treatment of these problems.

The *orange chakra* is centred on the spleen, and influences the process of *digestion* and *assimilation*. Treatment involving these should be focused on this centre. The *yellow chakra* lies in the solar plexus, and treatment is centred on this chakra where there is disharmony present in relation to *adrenal glands, pancreas* and *liver*. The *green chakra* is the heart. Diseases of the *heart*, the *blood* and *circulatory system* are treated through focusing on it. The *blue chakra* relates to the throat and is found at the back of the neck. Diseases to do with the *throat, thyroid* and *parathyroid glands* are treated via this chakra.

Indigo is the *forehead chakra*; it is located between the eyebrows and correlates with the pituitary gland. This is the master controlling gland for the entire endocrine system. It has to balance the under- or over-activity of the other glands and so may become overworked. Diseases of the *brain, eyes, nose, ears* and *nervous system* are treated by focusing on this chakra.

The following suggestions for treatment are derived from authorities on colour such as S. G. J. Ousley, Gladys Myer and Roland Hunt.

Red Ray

This is the element of fire. Stimulating and exciting the nerves and blood, it releases adrenalin, activates the circulation of the blood and vitalizes the physical body. Being a powerful stimulant, it must be used with caution. It should never be used alone, but followed by green or blue. Contra-indications are inflammatory conditions, and emotional disturbances.

Anaemia

Red colour breathing will be important as well as drinking red-charged water. Foods should include fruits and vegetables listed under the red ray. Ousley, in his book *Power of the Rays*, suggests that red light should be administered with a colour lamp first to the soles of the feet and then on the red chakra at the base of the spine at a distance of about six inches. He suggests a progression of five minutes each on the soles of the feet, then the calves, knees, thighs and the base of the spine, finishing up with a few minutes of green or blue light.

Paralysis

In the first treatment or so, it is recommended by various therapists that yellow light should be used in order to help the patient reorientate his mental state, which is likely to be confused. Yellow should be directed to the patient either by thought or by lamps. Purple light should then be administered to the base chakra for 10 minutes. The same ray should be allowed to play lightly up the spine for about five minutes and then allowed to rest on the soles of the feet, on the knees and the legs for about 10 minutes. However these times vary with each individual and should be sensed by the therapist or tested by the pendulum.

Orange Ray

The orange ray strengthens the lungs, pancreas and spleen, enlivens the emotions and creates a feeling of well-being. This is a stimulating, warming colour, an anti-spasmodic, and can — like the red ray — be used for lack of vitality, and muscle spasms or cramps. A general diffusion of light should be given over the whole body, then concentrated on the solar plexus and the base of the brain for 10 to 15 minutes.

Asthma

Again the orange ray is the one to use, although it is more imperative than usual that correct breathing is practised and the exercise of breathing in the orange ray should be done faithfully every day. Deep breathing, in which the lungs are properly cleared using the deep muscles of the chest and stomach, is most important. Also the mental attitude needs to be positive and optimistic. Treatment is the directing of the orange ray onto the chest and throat for 10 minutes at a time. As improvement is shown, the blue ray directed to the throat for 15 minutes will be found to be helpful. The drinking of orange-charged water also helps the condition.

Bronchitis

This is not a condition which responds easily to treatment, particularly if the condition is a long-standing one. For treatment the orange light is focused on the stomach and abdomen for the usual 10 to 15 minutes, or longer according to the patient's need. Orange and lemon juice have proven helpful for this condition and should be taken regularly. Again colour breathing of the orange ray should be followed.

Faulty Elimination

This is a condition which may show itself in vertical ridging of the finger and toe nails, but sometimes exists unsuspected by the patient because there is no outward sign of ill health. However it does respond rapidly to the administration of the orange ray and the drinking of orange-charged water taken twice daily.

Epilepsy

This is not an easy condition to cure once the disease has become established. However, treatment is by the *blue ray* to the head and the drinking of orange-charged water daily.

Yellow Ray

Activates the motor nerves and generates energy in the muscles, stimulates the flow of bile, is good for the skin, psychologically it can get rid of depression. This is a positive vibration and acts on the nervous system, influencing the mental attitude and the bodily vitality. The solar plexus centre is the most critical of all for the vitalization of the whole body, acting as it does as an assimilator and distributor of energies to the other chakras.

Dyspepsia

This condition may be caused by either too much red or too much blue in the system. Distinction may be made by the fact that those who draw in too much red are usually thin, while those who draw in too much blue are usually fat and lacking in vitality. Deep colour breathing of the yellow ray and the drinking of yellow-charged water should be practised during the day. The solar plexus should be exposed to yellow twice daily for 30 minutes. The antidote to an excess of red is the blue ray, as this reduces the irritation and restores health.

Diabetes

With this condition the blood becomes impoverished. The yellow light should be directed in the solar plexus centre for 15 minutes twice daily and the yellow-charged water also taken twice daily. This reduces the formation of fat in the cells and allows the condition of the blood to return to normal. Treatment will be lengthy.

Flatulence

Treatment for this condition is basically simply the drinking of yellow-charged water slowly between meals.

Constipation

The yellow light should be directed to the stomach and abdomen for 20 minutes night and morning. Colour breathing of the yellow ray should be practised and small quantities of yellow-charged water taken between meals. Yellow is contra-indicated in acute inflammation, fever, over-excitement and heart palpitation. However, too much yellow can bring on diarrhoea, as it stimulates the flow of bile.

Green Ray

Ray of harmony and balance, it is nature's tonic and exercises a strong influence on the heart and on the blood supply. Green relieves tension, it stimulates the pituitary gland and builds muscle and tissue.

Heart Complaints: Blood-pressure

Most therapists are agreed that heart complaints originate in the emotional body and are often due to an excitable nervous system. Green light focused on the heart centre helps to harmonize and heal. Visualization of the colour emerald by the patient is of help too. For low blood-pressure the quality of light directed to the patient should be dark and treatment last for 30 minutes. In high blood-pressure, a pale green light should be used for the same length of time. Green-charged water should be taken and plenty of green vegetables included in the diet.

Headaches

Treatment of these should be by means of diffused light over the whole body. Response is usually rapid.

Blue Ray

This ray is cold and astringent in quality. It is a ray with antiseptic qualities. It controls the throat chakra and produces a calm, peaceful vibration. It is called for in any feverish or inflamed condition as it is the antidote to red. Contra-indicated for colds, paralysis, chronic rheumatism and hypertension.

Sore Throat

The blue light should be focused on the throat for 15 minutes and the patient asked to gargle with blue-charged water every two hours.

Hoarseness

The blue-charged water should be taken in small doses and the throat given treatment by the blue light for half-an-hour. Blue ray breathing will help if done on rising.

Goitre

Treatment is directing the blue light to the throat for half-an-hour and gargling with the blue-charged water as frequently as possible until the condition improves.

Fevers

In all fevers the blue light should be focused on the centre of the inflammation.

Palpitation

Small doses of blue-charged water, alternating with green-charged water, have been found to improve the condition.

Bilious Attacks

Blue-charged water taken every hour acts most effectively.

Colic

One ounce of blue-charged water taken every hour is beneficial for this condition.

Jaundice

Treatment is by a diffusion of blue light over the whole body. Small doses of blue-charged water also prove beneficial.

Cuts and Burns

Application of the blue-charged water will help to take away the pain and assist healing. Use of the blue ray stops bleeding.

Rheumatism

Where the condition is acute the blue light can be used effectively. Where the condition is chronic, the orange ray is called for.

Indigo Ray

Cooling, astringent and electric, it works on the parathyroid glands, but depresses the thyroid. It reduces bleeding and also affects the emotional and spiritual levels. One can get rid of obsessions with it. Its use is called for in diseases of the ear, eye and nose; it is also beneficial in the treatment of certain nervous and mental disorders. Can also be used in the treatment of lung complaints and stomach troubles.

Deafness

It has been found that this condition is often due to unhappiness and introversion in childhood — the child learns to go inward and shut himself away from others — so that an effort to be more outgoing once the complaint begins to improve often helps a great deal.

The indigo light should be directed to the ear, or ears, and colour breathing of the indigo ray practised night and morning. At the same time the ear or ears should be bathed with indigo-charged water once a day.

Cataract

There are two stages of treatment. In the first, indigo ray breathing should be practised and the eyes bathed with indigo-charged water. Cloths wrung out with the charged water should be laid on the forehead.

In the second stage of treatment, the indigo light is directed to the eyes and forehead for 30 minutes daily.

Inflamed Eyes and Ears

Inflammation of the eye can sometimes be due to digestive disturbances; in these cases both the blue and indigo rays can be directed to the face and the head.

Earache responds to treatment by indigo light and indigo-charged water should be taken twice daily.

Pneumonia

This is an excellent and speedy remedy for pneumonia. Treatment by indigo ray lowers the temperature and heals the lungs.

Mental Disorders

The indigo ray has been found to be effective in the treatment of mental disorders when the patient is violent and excitable. Where the patient is depressed and inert the orange rays give results.

Violet Ray

The violet ray depresses the motor nerves and the lymphatic and cardiac systems. It purifies the blood and stops the growth of tumour. It maintains the potassium balance in the body. It is used quite extensively in orthodox medicine, but it is a powerful and subtle vibration and acts on man's highest body so that its use is contra-indicated where the mind is retarded or undeveloped. It controls the pituitary body.

Nervous Ailments

The use of this ray is called for when the patient is under a great deal of stress and strain and is a highly-strung and creative person. The opposite colour, yellow, cheers and raises the spirits when depression sets in and can be used in these cases.

Colour breathing and the drinking of colour-charged water is also beneficial.

Insomnia

Treatment by violet ray can be most effective in combating insomnia, especially where the patient is highly-strung and sensitive. However, both the calm rays of the blue and the indigo light have been used effectively.

Mental Disorders

It may be found that the violet ray is more effective in treating excitable cases than the indigo ray mentioned earlier. The blue ray is also often found to have a calming and soothing effect on the brain and so is helpful in the treatment of mental disorders.

Eye Troubles

Treatment by the violet ray can often be as effective as the indigo and the same process of treatment is recommended.

Gem Therapy

Gem therapy, like colour therapy, homoeopathy and radionic practice, approaches healing from the same angle; that of treating the whole man with all his physical and subtle bodies which form the force field surrounding and vitalizing his physical vehicle.

In colour healing, sunlight or electric light and various other methods are used to heal the patient. In gem therapy the seven principal gems are the source from which healing proceeds.

Allied to the personal treatment given by gem therapy where the patient has to come to the healer, a new treatment has been developed called *teletherapy*. Discs are set with gems and rotated by a small electric motor. The gems' rays fall on the patient's photograph and this link acts as a receiver of the rays and a conductor to the patient of the healing qualities of the gems' rays. This has, of course, great similarity to the treatment given by radionic practitioners, where the healer has a snippet of hair, blood spot, or a photograph of the patient and broadcasts the homoeopathic remedy in the potency required.

Dr A. Bhattacharyya has a practice in Naihati, India, where he treats patients daily using gem remedies and treatment is also given by the teletherapy devices for reaching absent patients.

There is some difference between the colours of the gems used and the colours of the major rays used in colour healing proper; however both treat the chakras. The following are as described by Dr Bhattacharyya:

Ruby	Astrologically corresponding to the sun — cosmic red ray. It is recommended for heart diseases, circulatory problems, anaemia, loss of vitality, eye diseases and various mental troubles.
Pearl	Astrologically corresponding to the moon — cosmic orange ray. It is used for diabetes, asthma, gallstones, diarrhoea, menopausal difficulties.
Coral	Astrologically corresponding to Mars — yellow cosmic ray. Liver diseases, impure blood, high blood pressure, skin troubles, haemorrhoids, sexual diseases.
Emerald	Astrologically corresponding to Mercury — green cosmic ray. Weak, digestion, colic, cancer, skin

problems, hypertension, heart troubles and ulcers.

Topaz   Astrologically corresponding to Jupiter — blue cosmic ray.
Effectively treats any throat troubles, asthma, laryngitis, childhood infectious diseases, insomnia and shock.

Diamond   Astrologically corresponds to Venus — indigo cosmic ray.
It is used for treating eye problems, various forms of paralysis, enlarged spleen, epilepsy.

All these have other indications and only a few are given above. Two other gems are frequently used; the *onyx*, which carries the ultra-violet frequency and can be used for bacterial or virus infection, and the *cat's eye*, giving off the infra-red frequency used for skin diseases, headaches and indigestion.

CHAPTER SIX

HEALTH FROM NUMBERS AND MUSIC

It is only too obvious that good health is the basis for all the other happinesses which life can offer us, so in this chapter I would like to make various suggestions for maintaining good health.

Each number represents a certain part of the body. The day of the month on which you are born will give a clue to the physical condition, and assist you through knowing your health, strength, and weaknesses.

Number One

Corresponds to the head and lungs. For those born on the first, or with many ones in the name (see p. 82), there is often a tendency to an inferiority complex and illness can too often result due to the lack of opportunity to make use of original ideas. For number Ones, exercises in deep breathing are beneficial, even essential, to success. Remember in adding up to your birthdate, number Ones are also those born on the twenty-eighth or any number which reduces to *one*, for example, 2 + 8 = 10 = 1. Always reduce your birthdate to a single figure.

Number Two

Corresponds to the nervous system, brain and solar plexus. The physical body is sensitive and impressionable. Very affected by noise, hard conditions and coarse associations. The feelings are sensitive, the person easily hurt and this can lead to illness and poor health generally. Diet is very important to maintain good health. Periods of rest and relaxation in a harmonious environment are helpful.

Number Three

Corresponds to the throat, tongue, larynx and the organs of speech. Many Three people become ill due to emotional disturbances, the feeling of lack of popularity and a general worrying tendency about the self. It is advisable for number Threes to cultivate a less pessimistic attitude to life and to worry less about what others think of them.

Number Four

Corresponds to the stomach, the right arm and the upper right side of the body. Rich foods should be avoided as this causes high blood pressure and problems. One of the most enduring of numbers, but even their endurance can be worn down by long periods of hard work and worry. The Fours should avoid taking themselves and life too seriously, as this can lead to lack of energy and circulatory problems.

Number Five

Corresponds to the liver, gall bladder, the left arm and the upper left side of the body. With many people born on a Five day, overactivity, restlessness, inner dissatisfaction and critical states of mind bring nervous tension, the bane of the Five; this upsets the whole physical coordination. Fives are subject to accidents and physical hurts entailing long periods of convalescence.

Number Six

Corresponds to the heart, blood and skin. With many Sixes, heart trouble is likely to be organic, not the sudden heart attacks so often found today, these belong more to Fours and Fives. Domestic problems, the affairs of children and lack of love tend to bring about chronic conditions with many Sixes. Sixes need good planning in their domestic affairs and attention to diet.

Number Seven

Corresponds to the spleen, white blood cells and the sympathetic nervous system. These are selective people generally, but they need to be so regarding diet, and also periods of relaxation are necessary and escape from too public a life. Repression of the emotions and feelings often give poor physical health. The lower left side of the body and the left leg are often affected.

Number Eight

Corresponds to the colon, eyes and bowels. Nervous indigestion, nervous headaches and ulcers result from an over-active and intense way of living; ambition often drives the Eight too hard. Of all the numbers, the Eight has both the greatest endurance and the most ability to recover. Sport and relaxation keeps the body healthy.

Number Nine

Corresponds to the kidneys and generative organs, also diseases hard to diagnose, brought about by self-indulgence and wrong habits of living. Alcohol or drugs are taboo for the Nines. Good health depends upon not being too impressionable or living too much in the clouds. Their escapist tendency can often be their undoing.

Each number has its characteristic colour, according to its rate of vibration. Each of the numbers marks strengths and weaknesses, so a little care will help you maintain good health.

Number	Corresponding colour
1	Red
2	Orange
3	Yellow
4	Green
5	Blue
6	Indigo
7	Purple/Violet
8	Opal
9	Carmine

It should be noted that number nine is all colour, for it contains within it all other colours.

Using the above colour key you can analyse your name and discover your key colour vibration.

The main meanings of the character in relation to the numbers are:

Vibration	Number	Meaning
Red	1	Love and will power.
Orange	2	Constructivity and joy.
Yellow	3	Intellectual power.
Green	4	Self-control.
Blue	5	Faith and aspiration.
Indigo	6	Integration.
Purple	7	Transmutation of desires.
Opal	8	Understanding of life.
Carmine	9	Compassion

The relationships of the numbers to the letters are:

Numbers	Letters
1	AJS
2	BKT
3	CLU
4	DMV
5	ENW
6	FOX
7	GPY
8	HQZ
9	IR

This method for analysing your name was developed by the long-term research of Roland Hunt, a skilled colour therapist and teacher who has written several books on colour healing in which he develops this method of deciding what colours are actually missing or overdeveloped in the aura at the present time. For those who cannot use the pendulum effectively, i.e. cannot place complete reliance on their ESP, this can be an excellent method of diagnosis.

Roland Hunt says that the colour alphabet key shown above does not involve or require extra-sensory perceptions in the user. It is based on vibrational rapport in the colour scale. He states that he has found it most accurate in diagnosis.

The theory is this: the first names and surnames of the individual carry the numbers/colour symbol vibrations causing physical, emotional and psychological characteristics which are gradually deepened throughout life. When you are analysing an individual you must use only those names which the person is using at the time of the consultation.

If we look now at the various ray traits in detail we shall get a better understanding of the various attributions for each colour vibration.

Characteristics of the Rays

Red Ray:

Will power, gratitude-graciousness, truthfulness, compassion, forgiveness, persistence, courage, sense of goodwill, obstinacy, resentment, passion, brutality, jealousy, ruthlessness. The last six are negative attributes.

Orange Ray:

Constructivity, enthusiasm, joviality, enterprise, self-assurance, exhibitionism, flamboyance, discouragement, joylessness, despondency, destructiveness. The last four are negative attributes.

Yellow Ray:

Intelligence, intuition, ingenuity, decisiveness, optimism, awareness, reasonableness, flattery, sly exaggeration, sly shrewdness, deviousness, deception, craftiness, malice, vindictiveness, deep pessimism. The last nine are negative attributes.

Green Ray:

Self-control, humility, justice, generosity, cooperation, discrimination, caution, prejudice, suspicion, envy, lack of judgement, callousness, indifference, miserliness, sense of grievance. The last eight are negative characteristics.

Blue Ray:

Aspiration, devotion, reliability, stability, service, resourcefulness, tactfulness, diplomacy, sense of beauty, ambition, superstition, indiscretion, unfaithfulness, lack of trust, dullness, apathy, inertia. The last seven are negative.

Indigo Ray:

Integration, practical idealism, clarity of perception, fluency of speech, tolerance, intolerance, disorderliness, impracticality, lack of truthfulness, lack of consideration, forgetfulness, idolatry, separativeness. The last eight are negative.

Violet Ray:

Idealism, dedication, self-denial, intuition, artistry, sense of power, snobbishness, sense of superiority, self-esteem, arrogance, subtlety, manipulation, fanaticism, treachery. As you can see, even under this high ray there are ways of using the energies in a negative way.

In finding and listing the various characteristics associated with the rays corresponding to the letters of the name, the lacks can be seen and remedied. Balance, the essential ingredient of any healing, will return. Where there are lacks then this can be remedied by wearing some article of the missing colour. On a more permanent basis, an effort by the person to develop the missing characteristics will restore health more surely.

Let us take now a few examples to show how the name and colour/number correspondences show up a person's character even if only one ray quality is used. Take two names we all know well:

M	A	R	G	A	R	E	T		T	H	A	T	C	H	E	R
4	1	9	7	1	9	5	2		2	8	1	2	3	8	5	9

Here we have:

Numbers	Colour Vibrations
3 ones	Red
3 twos	Orange
1 three	Yellow
1 four	Green
2 fives	Blue
no sixes	Indigo
1 seven	Purple/Violet
2 eights	Opal
3 nines	Carmine

Here no one colour predominates, although there are three ones, three twos, and three nines. Overall, there is a fair balance. There is a capacity for leadership and the ability to make constructive decisions and to carry things through to completion. The three nines give great compassion, there is understanding of life and ambition (the two eights). She also has faith, aspiration, and idealism, and is self-denying and intuitive (sevens). There is an absence of the six, the indigo ray, so there is a danger of intolerance at times, particularly with people who are unable to grasp a situation or solution as quickly as she can herself. Her greatest strength, that which makes her a great leader, is the fact that both her birthdate and her name number, if added and brought down to a single number, are the same. It is this single-minded approach which has made it possible for her to attain greatness.

Add name: 4+1+9+7+1+9+5+2 2+8+1+2+3+8+5+9 = 13/4

Add birthdate: 13.10.1925 = 13/4

If we now take the second well-known name we have:

$$\begin{array}{cccc} N & E & I & L \\ 5 & 5 & 9 & 3 \end{array} \qquad \begin{array}{ccccccc} K & I & N & N & O & C & K \\ 2 & 9 & 5 & 5 & 6 & 3 & 2 \end{array}$$

Translated, this becomes:

Numbers	Colour Vibrations
no ones	Red
2 twos	Orange
2 threes	Yellow
no fours	Green
4 fives	Blue
1 six	Indigo
no sevens	Purple/Violet
no eights	Opal
2 nines	Carmine

Here we are struck immediately by the large number of missing vibrations, which in some way certainly need supplying. The best way is to wear the colour or colours, but it is also helpful to concentrate on the colours which are missing. It is extremely important for someone who aims to be a leader to have the will power and stability to carry it through, and ones are lacking. Neil has no fours either (a lack of self control), and it is possibly this which makes the lack of love/will/leadership qualities more important than it would been had there been a four to balance things up. The lack of sevens may give overweening self-esteem and arrogance. The lack of eights intimates a love of power and position. However, all is not negative—he has intellectual ability and good reasoning power (two threes), and he can also be most constructive. There is a predominance of fives, a soul/mind colour, which will help to give resourcefulness, tact and diplomatic ability, as well as reliability, and stability to the nature.

His partnerships, including his marriage, will be very important to his career and success in leading his party, for he needs these to enable him to lead, as alone he has not the ability.

Add Name: $5+5+9+3 \quad 2+9+5+5+6+3+2 = 22+32+ = 9$

Add birthdate: $28.3.1942 = 11/2$

The nine contains all numbers so is clearly a dynamic plus, but the two works best in second place or in partnership.

Lacks and over-pluses point to imbalance, so these can be readjusted, as in this system of diagnosis you can see what needs doing. If a colour is missing this can be transmitted in various ways by using colour lamps, by colour-solarized drinks or by using the foods which correspond with the missing colours. Where the opposite is true and there is too much of a colour then a look at the diet can alter the colour balance. The tendency to such an imbalance will always be noted by the colour therapist and checked at each visit. Naturally, this method is only useful once and the checking must be done by the use of the pendulum, or if the sensitivity of the hands is developed these can be used to detect any weakness in the body. Some healers also use the hands to direct the visualized colour to the affected spot.

Music in Healing

Every sound emits a certain colour and takes on definite form. We have seen this recently on television, where colours emanating from music have been shown on the television screen. Every form also gives forth a sound, which is its key-note. Every created thing, from a molecule to a man and from the planet to the solar system, possesses a key-note of its own. The sum total of these notes makes up the music of the spheres. Everything pulsates to a definite rhythm, including the universe itself as it circles the sun; the planets too have their notes.

Flowers, trees and grasses have their own symphonic sound. In fact a delicate instrument has been perfected in Germany whereby the sound of growing grass can be heard. The winds and the waves have their own rhythm and the combined rhythms make up the key-note of the planet. Likewise man's organs all emit their own notes and make up the vital key-note of the individual. Max Heindel, a great German occultist, states that in health, the etheric body emits a sound which is like the hum of the bumble bee.

Since every object has its own key-note and overall blending of colours, it follows that upon entering a room one is immediately drawn to one person and repelled by another, often without a word being spoken. Where key-notes and colours harmonize there is understanding and affinity. Where they do not, the nerves are jarred and we say that so-and-so 'gets on my nerves'.

There are seven centres or *musical lights* which

correspond with the seven chakras and the seven-toned musical scale.

Music helps to develop these centres progressively and enables them to unfold their powers, so that the chakras visible to clairvoyant sight emit beautiful colours as they rotate continuously. The first centre becomes a luminous red, the second a reddish orange becoming gradually shot through with a soft green light, the third or solar plexus centre becomes irradiated with a pure gold light, the fourth, the cardiac centre, emits a luminous yellow and ethereal blue light. The fifth (throat centre), an azure blue, gradually becomes shot through with silver as the centre develops. The sixth (brow centre), when fully developed, reveals the colours yellow, blue and purple forming patterns of beauty. The seventh centre, in the dome of the head, when the body has been fully regenerated, emits a pure white effulgent light which blesses all who come within its rays.

There are healers who work with music as well as colour and it has been demonstrated that an unbalanced mind is particularly sensitive to musical vibrations, so that restful music can soothe the most excitable and violent patients. Conversely it might be said that pop records would excite already unbalanced or violent people.

The healing value of music has been recognized from earliest times. For instance, Paracelsus, a seer and therapist, prescribed certain compositions for certain maladies and practised musical healing. Today the power of discordant emotions to quickly or slowly destroy the physical body is much more understood, so that healing is not only directed at curing symptoms, but at reaching the seat of the disharmony in one of the subtle bodies, where such curative agents as music, colour, radionic treatment, homoeopathic medicaments and the Bach remedies can heal the whole man.

So back to music itself, and the fact that each one of us has a theme song which is formed from our names. Each number has its key-note on the musical scale.

Number	Letters	Key-note
1	AJS	middle C
2	BKT	D
3	CLU	E
4	DMV	F
5	ENW	G
6	FOX	A
7	GPY	B
8	HQZ	C (high C)
9	IR	D (high D)

Your 'Life Song'

If you understand music a little or are a musician, writing your 'life song' will cause you little trouble and in fact can be fascinating. You can use the chords of modern song writers to give it more charm. The numbers of the birthdate reduced to a single digit can be used to make a chorus. With each name a verse, the chorus can be the chords of the birthdate.

Your life song or musical key-note can be used to tune yourself to the purpose of your birth, and the playing of music which you enjoy and feel yourself attuned to can be the means of progressively unfolding the power of the centres or chakras. This tuning in to your 'life song' can be done either by singing or playing your key-note before meditation.

Frequent repetition of the chord of your own key-note can provide you with a wonderful system of protection against disease. It also has a soothing, harmonious effect on strained nerves or a tired body. The playing of this chord is also a wonderful way in which to lift the consciousness above the trials and difficulties of personal living and into the realms of inner knowing, where all is harmony and peace.

Astrological Applications

Those of you who are interested in astrology will like to know of the colour and musical correspondence inherent in your Sun sign and its relation to a particular part of the body. An illness is not always shown by the sign ruling the afflicted part. Sometimes it is shown equally well by the opposite sign, as the forces of the two signs intermingle in the body.

When the harmony of an organ of the body has been disrupted, disease is present until the rhythm and proper colour flow has been restored. The mind as a creative agent can heal the body, and to still the mind and quieten it so that it is better able to accomplish the healing of the physical body, it is best to play chords in the key of F and F sharp. The close affinity between opposite signs is shown by their musical relationship via their key-notes. Virgo and Pisces for instance, have Virgo C and Pisces B for key-notes.

The key-note of Aries is D flat, the colour of Aries is red. In astrological terms it rules the head and so the ear, eye, nose and all cranial nerves. Spiritually, Aries releases the highest impulses of the spirit.

Libra is its opposite sign, its key-note is D natural and its colour blue. A harmonic based on D will therefore release a spiritual force for the healing of afflictions of the head or kidneys.

Taurus has the key-note E flat, ruling the throat and organs of speech. The colour related to Taurus is green. These organs are destined to become the seat of power in the human body.

The opposite sign to Taurus is Scorpio, which rules the organs of generation and so holds the mystery of creation; its key-note is E. A harmonic based on E will, therefore, release a spiritual force for the healing of afflictions affecting the throat, larynx or the generative organs. The colour of Scorpio is deep red.

Gemini's key-note is F sharp, and Gemini rules the lower mind and the lungs, the vital breath, arms and hands. The colour of Gemini is yellow.

Sagittarius is its opposite sign, and its key-note is F. It holds the pattern of the higher mind, though it awakens the spiritual power and aspiration which gives it sway over the lower material mind. A harmonic based on the key of F will release the spiritual force for the clearing of afflictions of the mind and of the lungs. The colour of Sagittarius is purple.

Cancer's key-note is G sharp, and it rules the stomach and the breasts; through it awakens the faculty of intuition. Its colour is silver.

Capricorn is its opposite sign and rules the knees; its key-note is G, its colour black. This sign, using the key of G major, sends a ray of renewal to the earth. Therefore the key-note of Cancer is G sharp and that of Capricorn G natural. The key of G releases spiritual forces for the healing of diseases relating to the stomach, breasts and knees.

The key-note of Leo is A sharp and of its opposite sign — Aquarius — A natural. Leo rules the heart and the opposite polarity — Aquarius — the ankles and the circulation. The motivating power of Leo is love and of Aquarius mentality; their combination is said to be able to produce the superman of the Aquarian age. This is the union of heart and mind so difficult to achieve. The key of A releases spiritual forces for the healing of ills related to the heart, circulation and the ankles. The colour of Leo is gold and the colour of Aquarius blue.

The key-note of Virgo is C; Virgo rules the intestines and all their intricacies, its colour is brown, and its polarity is Pisces, whose sign rules the feet, the foundation of all understanding. The key-note of Pisces is B and its colour violet, its spiritual aim being the unity of all life. The keys of B and C major will release the spiritual forces for the healing of ills related to the intestines and the feet.

Sacred Temples

Colour and music work together to regenerate the body and these arts were used in the sacred temples of Egypt and Greece. Chants and invocations were spiritually constructed and so had powerful results. The priests taught the neophytes how to determine their key-notes, their sign and planet, and hereby gave them the ability to tune in on the planetary power. This wisdom and the use of colour, number and astrology all formed part of the teaching of the Mysteries.

The Persians celebrated the entry of the Sun into each zodiacal sign with the appropriate chants and music, stressing the vibratory key-note of the zodiacal sign and its ruler.

Music is indeed not only a healing and regenerative influence, but also one which enables the gradual unfoldment of man's spiritual powers through the raising of the vibratory level of the body and the clearing and stimulating of the chakras.

CHAPTER SEVEN

GENERAL INFLUENCES OF COLOUR

Colour plays a big part in our lives. Nature provides us constantly with varied shades. A bright blue sky can lift our spirits and a dark cloudy sky can make us feel low and depressed. Sunshine brings joy to most of us. Each season of the year has different colour hues. I do not have to talk about them, you all have experienced them in your own way. When the sky is clear at night and the moon is full, some people are influenced by it favourably or unfavourably.

Everything has a certain frequency of vibration, and that applies to all organs in the human body. If there is any deviation from the normal vibrations, it shows that the organ is not functioning properly. All organs have a vibration of their own, which can be detected, and it is the healer's job to wipe out these disease vibrations of the body and restore them to normal health. The application of the right frequency will alter the faulty vibration and bring the organ back to normal. Fatigue, strain, stress, fear and all negative emotions are culprits upsetting the healthy vibrations. Colour, being a pure vibration, when used in the right shade and focused on to the right place can correct the fault and restore the body to health.

Colour can be visualized with some perseverance. One can use these colours for self-healing or one can send them out to patients. Then, of course, colour can be used with help of a colour lamp. In my own practice I use a De La Warr colourscope regularly.

There are seven main colours in the spectrum: red, orange, yellow, green, blue, indigo and violet. The *warm colours* are *red*, *orange* and *yellow*.

Red is the element of fire and stimulates and excites the nerves and the blood. It releases adrenalin and stimulates the sensory nerves. It activates the circulation of the blood, excites the cerebro-spinal nerves and the sympathetic nervous system. It vitalizes the physical body, but because it is such a great stimulant it must be used with caution. Over-stimulation can be dangerous. Health means balance.

Red is contra-indicated in all inflammatory conditions and most emotional disturbances. One should never treat with red alone, but it should be followed either by green or blue.

Orange is a combination of red and yellow. It has an anti-spasmodic effect. It is good for the treatment of muscle-cramps and spasms. Orange aids the calcium metabolism and it strengthens the lungs, the pancreas and the spleen. This colour raises the pulse-rate, but it does not raise the blood pressure. It releases energy from the spleen and the pancreas. Orange strengthens the etheric body, enlivens the emotions and creates a general feeling of well-being, and cheerfulness.

Yellow activates the motor nerves. It generates energy in the muscle. It works favourably on the digestion, but if used for too long it might bring on diarrhoea, because it stimulates the flow of the bile. Yellow gets rid of parasites. It improves the skin and purifies the blood-stream. It activates the lymph. Yellow can depress the spleen. Psychologically it can get rid of melancholia and despondency. It is the colour of the intellect and of reason.

Yellow is contra-indicated in acute inflammation, delirium, diarrhoea, fever, over-excitement and palpitation of the heart.

Green is the middle colour of the spectrum. Green dilates the capillaries and produces a sensation of warmth. It relieves tension, but when used too much it gets tiring. It is a pituitary gland stimulant, and it is a muscle and tissue builder. Green is a disinfectant. Green loosens and at the same time regulates the etheric body and brings back the astral body which has suffered through shock, fatigue, illness or negative emotions.

Blue, *indigo* and *violet* are cooling colours.

Blue increases the metabolism. It promotes growth and suppuration. It heals burns very quickly. Blue is the colour of intuition and higher mental faculties.

Blue is contra-indicated for colds, gout, muscle contractions, paralysis, chronic rheumatism and tachycardia (rapid heartbeat).

Indigo is cooling, astringent, and electric. It works on the parathyroid glands, but depresses the thyroids. So when the thyroid is overworking, one treats the parathyroids with indigo. It purifies the blood-stream, and builds phagocites in the spleen. It reduces or even stops bleeding. When excessive bleeding is present, always treat the parathyroids with indigo. It depresses the respiration and is good for muscle toning. It has an anaesthetic effect when used too long. Indigo affects the vision, hearing and smell. It also affects the emotional and spiritual levels, and mental complaints with delirium tremens and insanity. One can get rid of obsessions with it, but in the latter case the healer has to protect himself, or herself as the case may be, in order not to pick the obsession up.

Violet depresses the motor nerves and the lymphatic system, as well as the cardiac system. It purifies the blood and is a leucocyte builder. Violet maintains the potassium balance in the body. It stops the growth of tumours. When treating cancer patients after they have had their operation three colours help:

Red to give energy to the system.

Green to stabilize the astral body.

Violet to restore the potassium-sodium balance.

Violet is a good and calming colour in cases of violent insanity. It controls excess hunger. It is a spiritual colour. The power of meditation is much deeper under violet light. The Comte Saint-Germain healed mostly with violet rays.

Ultra-violet is beyond the visible spectrum. It plays a very important part in the calcium-phosphorous metabolism. It fixes iron and iodine, therefore it is useful in the treatment of goitres and rickets. It normalizes the metabolism and glandular activities. It stimulates the action of the sympathetic nervous system and helps to ease pain. It acts favourably on the heart and on the lungs.

There are combinations of shades used in colour treatment:

Lemon, which is a mixture of a very light yellow and a very light green. Lemon rejuvenates the organism and throws out toxins. It is a laxative, eliminates phlegm, and strengthens the bones. It is a cerebral stimulant, activates the thymus gland, cures cretinism. It is antacid.

Purple and *scarlet*, which are combinations of red and blue. Purple is more blue and less red. Scarlet is more red and less blue. Purple has an analgesic property. It suppresses malaria, and it is a venous stimulant. Scarlet stimulates the kidneys and the sexual mechanism.

Magenta, a combination of red and violet, which energizes the adrenal glands and the action of the heart. It is a diuretic. In some cases it is an emotional stabilizer.

Turquoise, the opposite of the lemon ray, which builds the skin. When a burn is treated with blue, it might help to use the turquoise afterwards to hasten the skin formation. It is a cerebral depressant. It lowers mental over-activity.

Complementary Colours

Each colour has a complementary colour:

Red — Blue
Orange — Violet
Yellow — Violet
Green — Magenta
Blue — Red
Indigo — Orange
Violet — Yellow

Those who use the pendulum are at an advantage with regard to diagnosing, selecting the appropriate colour and fixing the duration of treatment. Patients should not only be treated for the illness they complain of, but they should be treated on three levels. For the illness on the physical level, then on the etheric level, which comprises the nervous system, and then on the astral, which comprises the ductless glands and the emotions. When one looks at the aura, most people can only see the vibrations of the three bodies just mentioned, for it is difficult to see the vibrations of the higher developed bodies. In the aura the physical vibration is always in a fixed position very near to the physical body. The etheric vibration is more or less always in near proximity, though it can look congested or as a double of the physical one, when it is in good health. The astral sheath is movable. It can be like a third layer, in a normal position, round the etheric, or it can be away from the body. In shock or emotional disturbances it moves from its normal position. After an operation the practitioner must first remove the anaesthetic toxins and then attend to the astral body.

Colour Vibrations of Some Foods

Red, *orange* and *yellow* foods have an alkaline effect.

Green foods are neither acid nor alkaline, they are neutral.

Blue, *indigo* and *violet* foods have an acid effect.

Red foods:	Meat, all red-skinned fruits and vegetables, beetroot, cabbage, cherries, peppers, grapes, onions, radishes.
Orange foods:	Carrots, oranges, pumpkins, sweet-corn, apricots, tangerines and peaches.
Yellow foods:	Apricots, butter, egg yolks, carrots, sweetcorn, grapefruit, mangoes, melons, marrow and yellow-skinned fruits and vegetables.
Green foods:	Green fruit and vegetables.
Blue foods:	Most blue fruits like plums, blueberries, bilberries, fish, veal, asparagus, potatoes.
Indigo foods:	These are the same as the blue and violet foods.
Violet foods:	Aubergines, purple broccoli, beet, purple grapes and blackberries.

Colour in the Home

When you plan to decorate a room think whether you want the room to look bigger or smaller.

Red, *orange* and *yellow* make a room look smaller, while *white*, *blue* and *indigo* make a room look larger. *Green* keeps it in the right proportion. *Blue* draws the ego and brings harmony with the environment. It brings the introvert out of his shell. *Red* makes a person egocentric, and *green* is very good on the cardiac circulation.

Colours of the Ductless Glands

So far colours have been mentioned only from the health angle. Now let us look into the colours of the ductless glands in relation to the planetary influence. If we consider the spiritual connection of the ductless glands with the latent potentialities, we find that they need different colours and much lighter shades. The spiritual colours of the glands are:

Dazzling blue	—	Pineal gland
Light yellow	—	Pituitary gland
Violet	—	Thyroid gland
Light golden yellow	—	Thymus gland
Golden yellow	—	Spleen
Blue	—	Adrenal glands

The *adrenals* are ruled by Jupiter.

When well aspected: benevolence, vision, optimism, courtesy, generosity, cheerfulness, religious understanding.

When badly aspected: over-confidence, extravagance, conceit, lawlessness, procrastination.

The *spleen* is ruled by the Sun.

When well aspected: vitality, courage, generosity, dignity, loyalty, faithfulness, parental instinct, leadership, responsibility.

When badly aspected: arrogance, overbearing and a domineering nature.

The *thymus gland* is under the love ray of Venus.

When well aspected: the individual develops the highest form of love, artistic ability, sense of beauty, cheerfulness, charm.

When badly aspected: sensuality, vulgarity, sentimentality, vanity, inconsistency.

The *thyroid gland* is under the rulership of Mercury.

When well aspected: dexterity, reason, intellect, thoughtfulness, good memory, studiousness, quick wit, eloquence.

When badly aspected: conceit, cunning, carelessness, lack of principles, gossiping, dishonesty, gambling, indecision, nervousness.

The *pituitary gland* is under the rulership of Uranus.

When well aspected: originality, love of liberty for all, independence, reformation, progression, intuition, mysticism, when in good harmony with a well aspected pineal-clairvoyance.

When badly aspected: eccentricity, fanaticism, irresponsibility, perversion, impatience, and, in some cases anarchy.

The *pituitary body* is the spiritual chain which connects Man with the highest vibrations of the Christ Spirit. The primary seat of this gland is the life spirit and the heart is the secondary seat. The colour of the life spirit is yellow. The pituitary is closely connected with the mystic path which leads to perfect initiation. The arousing of the pituitary body into action is one of the most important accomplishments in the development of the powers of the spirit.

The *pineal body* is ruled by Neptune. Neptune rules the spiritual side of the pineal, but Mercury rules the intellectual level. When Neptune is not well aspected the individual does not only deceive others, but himself as well.

When well aspected: contact with the super physical, inspiration, clairvoyance, prophecy, devotion, occultism, divinity, philosophy.

When badly aspected: delusion, morbidity, unreality, obsession, intrigue, black magic, a chaotic mental condition.

This does not mean to say that all the traits mentioned are in each individual, but some of them are in all of us.

The *spiritual side* of Man is represented by the *pituitary* and the *pineal glands*, the *personality* by the *adrenals* and the *thymus*, and the *link between them* is the *thyroid gland*. It is much easier to improve on the physical vibrations and on the emotional ones, than on the spiritual ones. Not only desire of the individual is necessary, but the person's Karma also has to be considered. If the person in question can visualize the colour, the improvement is quicker than when it is sent out.

CHAPTER EIGHT

HEALERS AND COLOUR

Colour healing has its practitioners all over the world and some startling work has been done both in the diagnosis of disease and its treatment.

In the USA we find D. P. Ghadiali, whose work and theories were discussed in Chapter One. He teaches the treatment and cure of disease through the application of colour.

Another great colour practitioner in the USA is Dr Francis J. Kolar of Los Angeles. He tells us that certain colours have healing qualities which rejuvenate our bodies and eliminate disease. A fellow practitioner, Audrey Kargere, in her book *Colour and Personality* (Weiser, 1980) gives a description of Dr Kolar's work in performing bloodless surgery. First he uses colour in order to induce hypnosis. Then he performs operations which remove fibroid tumours and crystalline deposits without incision or pain and with the patient remaining in normal consciousness. He can also produce insensibility to pain by means of coloured lenses or glasses which the patient wears. The lens of one eye is of a different colour from the lens of the other eye. An electric light bulb is held about two feet above the head of the patient and he is asked to look into it through the glasses to the count of ten, then he is told to close his eyes for the same count. He continues doing this and becomes quite insensible to pain, although he is conscious and able to converse intelligently with those around him.

In this way delicate operations can be performed, no special preparations are necessary, and there are no after-effects from the use of colour anaesthesia. Dr Kolar thinks that it is more difficult for the patient to recover from ordinary anaesthesia than from the actual operation. The principle behind this treatment is that correctly prescribed colours promote the attunement to the higher bodies and people are not aware of their physical bodies when perfectly attuned to the higher bodies. In fact, people who have developed colour consciousness are able to withdraw from pain. It seems that through the use of colour we can slip from body to body, or from plane to plane; this is indeed the secret of power. Dr F. J. Kolar's colour lenses induce this separation of the finer bodies. The conscious entity is isolated. This could be the key to future success.

An organization concerned with colour healing is The Aquarian Mystical Institute, founded by the late Ivah Berg Whitten.

In Britain one of the foremost healers is Theo Gimbel, a great master of colour, a teacher and a very dedicated soul. He lives in Gloucestershire. I am told he has some really stunningly beautiful colours. He runs conferences and courses on the use of colour.

Then there is Vicky Wall, who has developed the new Aura-Soma Balance cosmetic oils and many other things too. *Aura* refers to the magnetic field around the body. *Soma* refers to the being who resides in the body. *Balance* refers to bringing ease to the system through a natural method of restoring the whole body to health. Aura-Soma represents a therapeutic colour collection containing the trinity of colour, herbs and crystal energies. I shall give a more detailed description of the theory of this type of treatment later in this chapter.

Marie Louise Lacey is another of our modern colour healers. She lectures, has slides and various coloured oils for healing. I understand she links up oils and numerology most successfully.

Alice Howard is one of our really dedicated colour healers. She does not seek publicity or large material rewards, but over at least 25 years she has been giving unstinting service to her patients using both colour and homoeopathic remedies. She works with the pendulum to diagnose the malaise, the treatment and the length of time it should continue. It would be extremely hard to find someone as gifted and as dedicated to her life's work as Alice Howard. I am one of her most grateful and appreciative patients and I am happy to be able to register my eternal thanks for all she has done for me, my family and my friends.

More about these healers later.

The Universal White Brotherhood, whose teacher until recently was the Master Omraam Mikael Aivanhov, teaches that light is a living spirit and that the sun is the centre of the universe, the representative of the Holy One within view of earth, although not strictly on earth. One of the teachings for healing is to visualize oneself covered in a golden light. This can also be done for friends or relatives who need healing.

The teaching of the Brotherhood reminds us that light can be used in the most remarkable ways. Ancient civilizations such as Atlantis made use of light by catching and concentrating it with the aid of huge crystals and this solar energy ran all sorts of machines. In the twentieth century the laser has been perfected to give off an intense light. It is a physical symbol, designed by scientists, of the caduceus of Hermes, the wand or rod representing the spinal column and containing within itself both the positive and the negative. So the use of light and colour to heal is not new; it was in use in the Atlantean, Egyptian and Greek civilizations of ancient times.

Today the teaching of this great Universal White Brotherhood stresses that it is only through light and its various uses that we can transform ourselves and our world. Its literature is distributed through Prosveta Ltd, 4A St Helena Terrace, Richmond, Surrey, TW9 1NR, UK.

So we see there have been great teachers in the twentieth century giving out light to the world. If all the world has not listened, this is because people's vibrations have not been high enough to listen and accept, for as you know like attracts like. Everyone has to keep up the growing and developing process, moving from one level of enlightenment and understanding to another, but linking this well with past understanding. The truths which these great teachers have been giving to us is that Spirit exists, or perhaps we should say The Spiritual exists, the Holy One, and it is within a great plan for all that we are held and can respond or not according to our understanding and present growth. We have to try and keep our health even in hard times, for the hard times are the tests which the soul has to meet without giving up.

The *Balance* which is so important for health is found in the spine, which contains both the feminine and masculine elements and is so well expressed in the medical symbol of the caduceus of Hermes. In order to gain better understanding of health and healing we need to go back to the teachings of Pythagoras on the heart/balance energies, in fact to a more spiritual science, where living is seen as an opportunity to gain perspective, experience and so greater awareness all the time. Rudolph Steiner, another great teacher of the twentieth century, said, 'Do not regret mistakes or faults of the past, look forward to the next opportunity when you can actually meet a similar situation with more consciousness and with it avoid the previous mistake. Mistakes are in fact growing experiences and we learn much by these.'

It is said that symbolically we develop in the form of a spiral, each level higher than the last. Theo Gimbel says our difficulty is that we fail to face the challenges at some lower level and so build up some sort of resistance to that particular type of challenge, become obsessional about it and shape up a habit or pattern to deal with it, so that the flow is not a spiral but a circle, somewhere where we are imprisoned in the difficulties of the past and continue round and round in a prison of our own making wondering why our health is so poor.

Another factor which has much to do with general health is the form of architecture prevailing at any given time. Chartres, the spiritual school from 1280 to 1350, was the most powerful spiritual centre in Europe. Thomas Aquinas who taught there was able to translate the secrets of the Greek temples and use their healing for those who came for help. The sacred geometrical designs were incorporated into the cathedral at Chartres. These designs were also incorporated into the first Steiner school of spiritual science, which was burnt down in 1922. The second, built out of concrete, still at Dornach in Switzerland, is not quite so perfect in its geometrical designs as the earlier building. These are designs for healing and the Prince of Wales is so right to query some of the inhuman stuff being turned out today. Maybe we should go back to Pythagorean principles to be able to enjoy today's architectural offerings and of course benefit in our mental and physical health.

Theo Gimbel has an interesting background, as his father used to work with Rudolf Steiner. Through this he imbibed a good knowledge of Steiner's principles and was able to incorporate them into his own studies and research. This helped in the setting up of the Hygeia studios, a centre for therapy, teaching and research.

Both Steiner and Gimbel divide colours into eight main ones plus black and white. Here we consider them in the environment as we live with them.

Blue

Most of us need blue today as there is so much stress around and we need the cool, calm, relaxing atmosphere which it gives.

Orange

This is a warm colour containing both red and yellow. It protects from the extremes of red and yellow on their own. It is a good colour for many rooms. In treatment it can be used for lethargic conditions.

Orange is the complementary colour to blue. People are encouraged to breathe out in the blue room, to exhale. A feeling of release is created. So blue is a great help in all cases where tensions and restrictions in the ordinary environment have produced ill health. Blue helps asthmatic conditions, as tensions help to produce this situation. Blue is reinforced by the use of orange. A balance must be achieved between blue and orange or red. This can be achieved by the use of the various colour healing lamps with their choice of filters.

Red

I have said before, a little of this colour goes a long way, whether this is viewed from either the psychological or the physical angle. A great deal of red in the decoration makes the room look smaller and also stimulates the inhabitants too much. If it is the ceiling which is painted red people develop a feeling of oppression, even become claustrophobic. A little of the colour gives warmth, a feeling excitement and stimulation.

The complementary colour is turquoise. Physiologically, the red light or decoration raises the pulse rate, inhaling is stimulated and this is good if there is a sluggish condition to be healed. Paralysis is influenced by this colour and a rhythm of blue/red or red/green could be set up which would be beneficial in such cases.

Yellow

This is a lovely, bright, glorious colour like sunlight, to which it is akin. Everyone needs the sun. Imagine lack of sunlight for any length of time — the crops would not ripen, the flowers would not bloom and the people, children and adults would be rather depressed. Yellow is a delicate colour and does not stand well on its own as it needs the protection of green or orange, to which it can change easily. It is a colour which affects mainly the mental side of man. Its impact in this area can either be one of loss of anchorage or of direction. Hence it is not recommended for use by itself when driving! To live in a pure yellow environment would not be helpful.

Yellow seems to unbalance people and removes their control so that they tend to act irrationally and abandon their feeling of responsibility. Violence can be sparked off by yellow light so it is to be hoped that centres where there are discos or acid house parties do not sport yellow walls. If a room has yellow lighting it is quite all right provided there are plenty of furnishings and objects around the room bringing it down to earth.

Violet is the complementary colour.

Green

Used as decoration in a room it is rarely successful, for it gives people a feeling of deprivation. This may be because in nature green is the next stage to decay.

Violet

Composed of blue and red, it gives a feeling of shelter, it is relaxing and also stimulating. It gives the ability to concentrate and so is a good colour for meditation. Violet light in healing has a gentle contracting effect, good for infected areas of the body.

Green is the complementary colour and turquoise too.

Turquoise

This colour has much of the coolness of blue; it is calming and soothing. Too cool and detached for living.

Red is the complementary colour.

Magenta

A mixture of red and violet. It is a very spiritual colour according to both Rudolf Steiner and Theo Gimbel. Magenta-coloured light would lift us to a realm beyond the physical. Gimbel states that with a violet decor it could act as a primaeval and futuristic death and rebirth situation. It should only be used by people experienced in the colour field as it is the most powerful of all the colours. It holds past and future and so can introduce deep healing possibilities. Gimbel says it has such a high quality of healing power its use might be described as an experience of excarnation, when the spirit frees itself of the physical. He thinks that in very rare cases its use might help to clear away accumulated darknesses which have helped to clog up the filters which give Man access to the spiritual world.

Black

Black is the extreme. When this colour is chosen in the colour test mentioned earlier, then the situation is pretty grim. It is limitation, the end, when the physical world goes over to the invisible, the spiritual. In the colour scale it stands at the end of red and the beginning of violet. Magenta arises out of it as a phoenix from the dead.

White

All is excluded from white. It is purity as a non-experience. Both black and white hold the total potential within.

Brown

Brown can be the colour of help, service, sacrifice. The colour of autumn leaves.

Colour can also be used to affect plant growth beneficially. Peter Tompkins and Christopher Bird have done a lot of research into plant life and described their investigations in a book called *The Secret Life of Plants*. Theo Gimbel has done experiments along the lines of plant growth with the use of colour and music and in both cases the plants have done very well. Dr E. F. Schumacher, in a book called *Small is Beautiful*, tells us that plants respond to tender loving care as do humans and that if too few people are tending a fruit tree, the tree will bear little fruit.

It is possible that somewhere sometime, someone will use music and colour to improve animal growth. It is unlikely that this will be altruistic, i.e. for the sake of the animals and their welfare, but will simply be a wheeze to get more money from the growth of the animals.

Aura-Soma Colour Therapy

A new form of colour therapy, its essence was received in meditation by Vicky Wall, ex-apothecary and practising therapist for 40 years.

The word *aura*, as we already know, refers to the colours seen by clairvoyants which surround every person, i.e. their magnetic field. These physical auric colours relate to the chakras, the vibratory wavelengths found in the spinal column. The word *soma* is derived from the Greek meaning 'body'. So *Aura-Soma* is all about holistic healing, the healing of the body, mind, and spirit. It does not treat just symptoms. Aura-Soma is all about regenerating, revitalizing and rebalancing the human aura. By feeding back the appropriate colours, Aura-Soma restores the balance, enabling the body to resume its normal rhythm.

Therefore, this system could have no other name but *Balance*. Based on beauty oils, healing herbs and aroma essences, it is a unique method of restoring the whole. Beauty is not just skin deep and many disorders and blemishes are merely the outer manifestation of inner disturbances.

Vicky reminds us that researchers throughout the centuries have acknowledged the profound influence of colour upon our physical, mental, emotional and spiritual well-being. Each colour component of light has its own vibratory wavelength and specific qualities of energy capable of affecting the whole gamut of human emotions. For example, blue is a peacemaker. The influence of colour is reflected in our everyday thinking and speech. Colour is also medically recognized as an antiseptic and healing agent, e.g. gentian violet, magenta paint, crystal green, etc.

Vicky Wall goes on to explain to us the basis of her healing therapy, saying that the human aura is not only a consistent specimen of colour from red at the base of the spine to violet at the head, but that each colour has important therapeutic effects. Red appears to govern the reproductive area and to impart a strong physical energy to the circulation. Yellow seems to be connected with the digestion, liver and pancreas. Green is linked to the heart and lungs. Blue is centred in the throat. Violet at the top of the head has an effect on the whole body via the pituitary gland of the endocrine system and, like ultra-violet, has a healing effect in inflammatory conditions.

Therapy and Diagnosis

Oils (known as *Balances*) are used in Aura-Soma therapy. These consist of pairs of oils that form upper and lower layers within a set of bottles. A few personal details are taken from the patient and then they are asked to choose a Balance. The patient selects four bottles. The selection is the revelation of the person. It is important to observe the colours that are not present, for these give insight into what the client prefers *not* to look at.

The first bottle represents the aura, the past, the beginning of the soul's spiral through timelessness co-creating its programmed pattern to the present and thus into the future. The first bottle is the life lesson and the life purpose.

The last bottle selected represents the present and the future. These, the first and the last choices, should coincide in variation and subtlety, for the past is part of the present. If this does not occur, the client should be encouraged to make further selections until this is achieved. When there is no matching between the first and the fourth bottle it can indicate a pocket of resistance. The last selection is the 'key' that opens the gate to the full knowledge and healing of the person. The key is that which correlates the past with the present.

The second and third choices indicate the progress and development through time of the purpose and the mission.

Readings are taken on three levels so that a complete picture gives in-depth perception into the client's story. Aura-Soma is rare among therapies in that it is a process of non-interference, a non-intrusion whereby the patient 'selects' his/her own treatment through that which colours his life and looks into the true mirror of self, recognizing the deep need within.

There are many methods of colour therapy which use colour through light or the exposure of the body to filtered colours, as already mentioned. These are used in Aura-

Soma therapy too, but the difference between this and other colour therapies is that the oils can be applied to the skin, which absorbs the colours, essences and extracts safely, thus affecting mind, body and spirit through the aura as well as on a completely physical level.

The rhythms of the healthy body are dependent on the condition of the aura and the chakras. Aura-Soma regenerates, revitalizes and rebalances the aura by replenishing the colours which have become weak. It also restores the body's natural immune system.

Each colour has a sympathetic resonance with a particular part of the body as listed below:

Colour	Chakra and Physical Area	Other Influences
Violet	Crown/top of head	For and of the spirit, cooling.
Indigo	Brow/pineal	For inspiration and intuition/cooling.
Blue	Throat/base of skull	Specific healer.
Green	Heart, chest, shoulders	Harmonizing, relaxing.
Yellow	Solar plexus, middle of back, kidney	Wisdom ray, affects lower mental and the emotional bodies, cleansing and heating.
Orange	Navel/spleen, abdomen and small of back	Imparts vitality, strengthens etheric body, heating.
Red	Base of spine/ reproductive organs	Physical, wilful and assertive, heating and for losing weight.

This is an interesting method of attempting holistic healing for it does not just deal with the physical symptoms of disease presented by the patient or uncovered by him/her in choosing the bottles (Balances), it also has subtler meanings.

The true aura, the Higher Consciousness, that which continues its spiral from the beginning, through eternity, contains its own personal record and, as fingerprints are the identity kit of the person, so the aura is the identification of the soul essence. All previous experiences from the beginning of time leave their mark upon the true aura. Indeed to a clairvoyant gifted in this way, the aura itself is a map, a record of the true personality and imparts the complete soul sense and recognition of one for another. In fact, it is through the aura recognition that one old soul recognizes those with whom he or she has travelled in the past, in other lives. Thus twin souls meet and recognize one another instantly.

Besides the therapy there are many other substances on offer, such as all-purpose skin cream, skin-revitalizing lotion, beauty bath and pomander, said to be the essence of Aura-Soma. For more information on Aura-Soma, see Vicky Wall's *The Miracle of Colour Healing* (The Aquarian Press, 1990) or contact Dev Aura, Little London, Tetford, Lincs, LN9 6QL, UK.

Hygeia Studies

Theo Gimbel set up the Hygeia Studios in 1968 after 12 years of part-time research. He directs weekend seminars there relating to colour, sound, and form. He was born in Germany in 1920 and educated at the Rudolph Steiner school in Basle. Later he came to England to pursue a course of study in curative education and was awarded the Diploma of Curative Education. He has worked for some years with mentally-handicapped children and also with prisoners. It was during this time that he became aware of the significance and effect that colour and form had on children under his care. A small incident will show the importance of the environmental factor in treating mental illness and emotional disturbance.

The two children of clients were disturbed by their parents' divorce. Theo Gimbel designed a room where the corners were so smooth that their fears could not conjure up imaginary devils lurking in corners, and at the same time the room was done out in cheerful but soothing colours. The main problem, Theo explained, was to restore the children's sense of security.

The weekend seminars at Hygeia Studios are attended by lay people, medical staff, educationalists and many others interested in a new approach to wholeness of mind, body and spirit. Theo says in his brochure, 'research and teaching became an essential part of our work.'

The studios are a centre for research into the basic principles of colour, form, sound and movement, and with the help of researchers Theo has developed the colour wall and the colour level lamp. More and more people are becoming aware that these principles have far greater effect on human well-being than has hitherto been known.

Theo Gimbel's work has covered research on behalf of hospitals, nursing homes and other environments where individuals can benefit from this very advanced application of design. The studies are unique in the research they are carrying out and they can, and do, provide invaluable assistance to existing medical services. Maybe a link here between one type of healing and another?

The courses offered consist of lectures, practical work, demonstrations, teaching and cultural activities such as concerts, poetry and drama. They sound attractive, provided you are vegetarian, don't go in for drugs, and also like meditation, which is quoted as taking place at 8.00 a.m. and 10.00 p.m. daily throughout the course.

Practical Advice for the Colour Healer from Theo Gimbel

Naturally you will want as harmonious surroundings as possible, so the colours and furnishings will be important.

A tremendous amount will depend upon your warm and welcoming attitude to the patient. Make him very quickly feel at home. Probably the best advice is to listen very carefully. When in doubt, consult those who have been in practice longer than you and cultivate your intuition.

Always let the patient know what your diagnosis is; uncertainty is always bad for the person as it is likely to cause stress. If you find it difficult to communicate something then address yourself to the patient's Higher Self once the person has left the room. This will not be a vain effort — the response will come back to you at the person's next appointment. They may even broach the difficult question themselves and so you will be spared further embarrassment. Most therapists will work with the pendulum to ascertain diagnosis, treatment and the length of time it should be continued.

For the therapy room itself, the floor should be of wood, stone or cement. Plastic tiles or nylon carpets are not advisable. The carpet should be blue, turquoise or lilac. The walls should be cobalt blue, with the ceiling of a lighter colour and the lights on a dimmer switch. The design of a figure of eight should be included in the ceiling design as a protective element.

A cubicle to undress in should be provided and a basin and water, also a white garment for the patient to change into before the healing session. This allows any colour to be used without the dress interfering with the colour treatment.

Most therapists will use a colour ray lamp into which the various coloured filters can be fitted. Then the rest of the room can be left in a pale blue light. Either direct or indirect help re getting a colour healing lamp can be obtained from the Hygeia Studios, Brook House, Avening, Tetbury, Glos, GL8 8NS, UK.

Do keep notes on each patient with the dates of appointments and the treatment given. Some of you may like to play tapes of healing, restful music during a session.

Use your intuition or the pendulum to decide if music should accompany the treatment and then, with your pendulum, choose one which will be suitable for the patient. Always ask for God's help in this healing and ask that you may be the channel for that help if it is God's will that it should be so. Use your pendulum to decide on the length of time the treatment should last.

Of course there may well be changes in the courses, in their requirements and whole structure as time goes on and what may be true today can change completely tomorrow as research continues.

Theo designs interiors and colour schemes for hospitals, clinics, schools and the occasional private home. He has also developed instruments for use in hospitals to help the staff restore health. He makes a psychological study of the people who are living or going to live in the houses and so applies colour and form to suit them and keep them healthy.

Among the instruments he has designed is a colour level lamp MK1. It is easy to control the lamp for healing by adjusting a few knobs. The colour and light can be varied and enable the practitioner either to stimulate or relax the patient. The design of the lamp is very much inspired by Steiner's ideas.

Theo is a natural healer; he does laying on of hands and reads auras, combining this with his colour theories. He puts much emphasis on the spine in healing for we have to remember the spine is the balancing factor in the body. If the spine is healthy then the rest of the body is likely to follow suit.

The Atlanteans

Other healing groups involved in the use of colour are the Atlanteans. This is a group who base their philosophy on the occult traditions of Atlantis. They originally started off in London, but have now expanded, and their activities are based in Cheltenham, Bristol and Bromley. They are of interest, for occult healing is part of their work and there are classes to train members in the use of their minds to project healing colours. Unlike the radionic experts they do not use instruments, but simply their mental and visualizing powers to direct the colours through their hands and so to the patient. The mind is considered to be the creative and healing agent and energy follows thought.

Alice Howard

Alice Howard studied psychology in Vienna and works now in research into homoeopathy, biochemistry and allied healing methods which are collectively known as fringe medicine. She is also a practising colour healer and belongs to the Radionic and Homoeopathic Associations, and to the British Society of Dowsers.

She started out as a water diviner, later going over to radiesthesia, radionics and colour healing. The difference between radionics and radiesthesia is that the radiesthetist uses the pendulum or rod and the radionic therapist uses diagnostic and broadcast instruments.

Alice told me that colour can be sent out mentally or with the help of an instrument, a fact that we have already mentioned earlier. She herself works with an actual colour instrument, a colourscope, made by the De La Warr laboratories at Oxford, which focuses on the organ that is in disharmony. She is able to insert colour slides according to the patient's need. On the back of the instrument are dials which make it possible to focus onto the right organ. By directing the chosen colour she is able to correct the bodily imbalance. She stressed that it is much better if the disease is not treated purely on the physical level, for imbalance in the mental or emotional levels affects the physical and manifests in the body itself, but does not originate there.

Mrs Howard diagnoses through her pendulum and as she said, it must be understood that the pendulum does not give a person knowledge which is unknown to them. She stressed that the therapist must know the relevant subjects well in order to ask the right questions and so get the right answers. The pendulum only answers yes or no, or indicates the level of activity of any given organ in the body. She gave a rather horrifying list of the subjects an expert in colour or radionics should know, and these included psychology, anatomy, physiology, pathology, and bacteriology. All these subjects has, as she stressed, relevance at different times in her practice.

She also reminded me that successful diagnosis with the pendulum depends upon being gifted with a strong ESP faculty and that, as in everything else, practice makes perfect, provided the faculty is there to start with.

Naturally it is essential to diagnose before treatment is started because it is no good treating symptoms alone; one has to find out the underlying cause.

For instance, if there is a malfunction of the liver, it is essential to find out whether it is an acquired or inherited weakness. If it is inherited, the illness has to be removed by treating the base chakra, mostly with the green ray, but occasionally other colours are needed as well. If it is not inherited, then one has to establish the cause of the weakness — whether it is a virus infection or just functional trouble.

Length of treatment varies. The first treatment must be fairly short as otherwise too much colour all at once would be a shock to the system. The next treatment varies in length but this can be established by the pendulum. It usually takes three-quarters of an hour.

As to results, Mrs Howard tells me that she has had excellent results with nervous troubles, asthma and liver trouble. She finds that arthritis and sinus trouble are often difficult to clear. Skin troubles too, unless they are occupational. Skin troubles are often inherited and also involve the nerves, the digestive system and the whole emotional outlook.

Cancer patients have to be referred to a surgeon in the first instance, but after an operation colour can definitely remove any remaining cancer toxins. In this respect Alice Howard feels that early diagnosis before the disease manifests in the physical body is more than advisable.

Like most fringe medical treatments, colour can be given by personal or absent treatment, the latter through the patient sending the healer a witness, which may be a bloodspot, a photograph, or a hair snippet. Mrs Howard often has quite an array of photographs and other items under treatment at any one time.

Lastly, she had something interesting to say about colour treatment and habits. She mentioned that it was difficult to remove disharmonies in the physical body when what lay behind these were habits of behaviour very deeply ingrained in the subconscious, often leading to compulsive or obsessive actions. First of all the ingrained habit has to be attacked. Sometimes in this respect there can be simply a deeply-rooted pattern of behaviour, but sometimes there is an actual obsession by an entity such as is mentioned in the Bible. She wanted me to stress that she is not an exorcist but a colour healer, and she uses the colour advocated for this in the rate book, the technical book which goes with the colourscope. She will not treat obsessions personally, but only by sample and absent treatment.

Marie Louise Lacey

Marie Louise Lacey is an accomplished therapist and a member of the Association of Colour Healers. We met a few years back when she came to address the Society of which

I was conference secretary. She introduced us to the Aura-Soma colours after her lecture. She has recently written a book, *Know Yourself Through Colour* (The Aquarian Press, 1989) which includes a pack of 28 colour cards the reader can use to clarify what is happening in their life and to make the best of opportunities in the future.

Electronic Gem Therapy

This is a most interesting therapy which has burst upon the scene at a most appropriate time when many of the major planets are in earth signs. This energizing system uses the fruits of the earth, crystals and gemstones. It is therefore in harmony with the forward thrust of evolution and so will prosper in helping humanity.

Jon Whale, an inventor, engineer and mystic, conceived the idea for an electronic caduceus whilst in a state of high consciousness and has spent the last six years transforming his vision into reality. Gems are an inexhaustible source of energy which can be used to heal, balance, invigorate or tranquilize in a completely natural way. The caduceus uses high-frequency vibrations to release the energy rays of gems. The equipment is adjusted above the body so that each particular type of gem radiates energy to the appropriate chakra.

The Story of the Caduceus

This is the staff of Mercury. Two snakes entwine up the staff seven times and the head of the staff has two wings fluttering from it. Carried by heralds and ambassadors in time of war, it has been adopted by the medical profession as their emblem.

Its origin is charmingly described in a Greek myth. Apollo discovered his herd of cattle was missing and accused Mercury of taking them.

At the throne of Jupiter, Mercury denied everything and produced his famous lyre. As Mercury played all the gods in Olympus held their breath with delight. Apollo was so impressed he said the music was well worth the 50 cattle. So pleased was Mercury with Apollo that he gave him his lyre. Apollo in return gave Mercury a golden wand called the caduceus, which had power over sleep and dreams, wealth, health and happiness.

The Electronic Caduceus

The electronic caduceus is an electro-mechanical version which enables etheric energy to be taken in through the seven chakras in the human body, bringing about increased energy, vitality and health. Seven different gemstone transducers are mounted along a support member. The subject may lie or stand in front of the caduceus to receive the energy output from the gems, which are excited and controlled by electronic apparatus.

Apart from the large Caduceus 7 Chakra Energizer, which can stretch across a couch, there are also three types of pocket instrument which balance and energize the electromagnetic fields of all living organisms by utilizing the natural energies that radiate from precious gemstones. They will easily induce all the desirable moods from sleep through to alertness, as well as tranquillize or stimulate selected parts of the body in a pleasant way. They can alleviate pain and treat various conditions. Gemstones are an inexhaustible source of energy, they have an immense healing capacity, and once acquired, their power does not run out. The gems are held in transparent cylindrical vials with screw tops (called gem transducers). These gem transducers clip into a holder that resonates the gems electronically. The energy that radiates from the gem transducers can be felt with the palm of the hand. Each type of gem has its own special property and feeling. The gem transducers are held in the hand and used like a wand to treat the parts of the body required. The output level can be easily adjusted, along with the vibrational rate. This, Jon says, is safe and simple to use, designed for the professional healer and therapist, yet so easy to use and understand that anyone can train themselves to use it for their personal healing.

I was able to experience the balancing of my own energies under the soothing rays of the Caduceus 7 Chakra Energizer and found myself rising up like Aphrodite from the foam, renewed and vital.

Jon has many recommendations from grateful clients all signed so that, as he says, you can see that these people are all different types from their handwriting, which is something in which he is also interested.

Jon is someone who has put in a great deal of painstaking research and has information on the what and how of healing by electronic gem therapy. Any questions which you have on his work he can surely answer.*

He has realized a dream in his invention which links electronic technology with the ancient teachings of Ayurvedic medicine about the human aura and the chakras.

You can see now that there are many new wonderful therapies which complement those already in existence and give a new slant as a new age is about to be born.

* He may be contacted at 290 Hanworth Road, Hampton, Middlesex, TW12 3EA, UK.

INDEX